A Guide To Understanding Alzheimer's And Other Dementias

Physiology, Perceptions, Communication, Stages, Grief and Death

Tam Cummings, M.S.
Gerontologist

You can reach Tam at tam.cummings@gmail.com.

© 2008 by Tam Cummings
All rights reserved.

Printed in the United States of America.

Acknowledgements

To Tammy L. Knott, thank you for your support, your encouragement and your friendship. I would not have completed this without you.

Joanne Johnson, CDP

Director of Sales and Marketing

703.994.4561
571.325.4792
571.665.2661

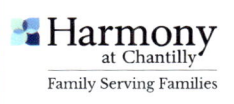

Harmony at Chantilly
Family Serving Families

jjohnson@harmonyatchantilly.com
2980 Centreville Rd Herndon VA 20171

Contents

Chapter 1	Defining Dementia Dementia versus delirium	Page	1
Chapter 2	History of Dementia Alois Alzheimer's discovery	Page	17
Chapter 3	The Four A's of Alzheimer's Amnesia, Agnosia, Aphasia and Apraxia	Page	27
Chapter4	Physiological Changes Normal Aging versus Dementia Aging Changes in the Brain	Page	45
Chapter5	Perceptions of Their World Visual, Hydration and Nutrition, Hearing, Tactile, Speech, Pain and Temperature	Page	54
Chapter 6	Communicating with Alzheimer's Patients Techniques for Communication	Page	75
Chapter 7	Global Deterioration Scale Characteristics Seven Stages of Dementia	Page	86
Chapter 8	The Grief Process Five Stages of Grief	Page	121
Chapter 9	Death and Alzheimer's The Process of Death	Page	129
Illustration	The Brain	Page	141

Chapter 1 – Defining Dementia

Defining Dementia

We get the word "dementia" from a French physician named Pinel, who in 1801 coined the word "demence." Pinel was writing about a client of his who had lost her memory and could no longer recognize herself or her family, dress, groom or feed herself, walk or speak. From the word "demence" we get the word "dementia."

Dementia is actually referring to any one or 48 or so different disease processes attacking the brain with a severe enough effect to impact social or cognitive functioning. Alzheimer's disease is actually one of the dementias, rather than a separate disease. It's not that a person has Alzheimer's or dementia; it's that a person has Alzheimer's and that is one of the dementias.

The disease processes of dementia may originate from different causes, but for many, the end result is a set of seemingly bizarre and confusing behaviors. These

Chapter 1 – Defining Dementia

behaviors which actually point to various stages of the disease and allow professionals and families to determine which lobes of the brain are being damaged or attacked. Think about the following examples:

In Maryland, 90-year-old grandmother of five leaves her home in the middle of the night, wearing a nightgown. She walks out into a snowstorm, only to be found the next day, frozen to death in a neighbor's yard. In Virginia, a daughter reports her deaf father is waking her up, night after night, to ask her to quiet the (invisible) woman singing in his room.

In Texas, an elderly couple drives to the local grocery store to shop and fail return home afterwards. Family members alert the police and the couple is found three days later in Arkansas, dehydrated and confused, more than 600 miles from home. In Ohio, a daughter describes neighbors calling to tell her that her 54-year-old mother is running down the street in the middle of the day, naked.

In California, police officers respond to a call from an elderly man reporting that his son is stealing his money and people are beating him. They arrive to discover the son calmly trying to reason his father into coming back into the house to finish his breakfast. In Florida, a husband reports his 70-year-old wife has suddenly picked

Chapter 1 – Defining Dementia

up a 30-pound floor lamp and swung it at a care giver, narrowly missing the care giver's head.

In Washington, a son receives a call from his mother's banker. She has paid the mortgage five times in one month.

The people and families mentioned above are all dealing with the effects of some type of dementia. Medically, dementia is a disorder characterized by the development of multiple cognitive impairments, including memory loss, that are directly related to a general medical condition occurring in the brain. The best known dementia is Alzheimer's disease, which now is estimated to account for an estimated sixty to eighty percent of the diagnosed dementia cases.

Currently in the United States an estimated 5.7 million people have Alzheimer's disease. Of those, it is believed only 2.5 million have been diagnosed with the disease. Of those 2.5 million, only 1.3 million are thought to be on medication for memory support. And sadly, a further breakdown of the 1.3 million seems to indicate that only 600,000 of those persons are actually on the correct medication.

It is important for persons dealing with this disease or their family members that proper medical attention is

Chapter 1 – Defining Dementia

sought. Medical persons trained to properly diagnose and medicate for this disease include geriatricians, geriatric psychiatrists and neurologists who specialize in dementia.

The "general medical condition" mentioned above varies based on the specific type of dementia, but it will usually involve an atrophying of the brain either in all lobes or in specific lobes. The type of dementia also determines the kind and frequency of damage is being done to the brain and the aggressiveness of the disease as it relates to an individual's decline.

The American Psychiatric Association's literature describes Alzheimer's as a "multifaceted loss of intellectual abilities, such as memory, judgment, abstract thought, and other higher cortical functions, and changes in personality and behavior."

Dementia however, should not be confused with delirium, which is also characterized as fluctuating memory impairment. Delirium causes the person to display a reduced ability to maintain attention and/or an inability to shift attention appropriately. The symptoms in dementia are more stable and unchanging, while delirium can be reversed and may be caused by common illnesses such as urinary tract infections or pneumonia.

Chapter 1 – Defining Dementia

One way to think about differentiating between the two is this: dementia means that over the past several months and years, there has been a progressive decline in Mom's memory and abilities, while delirium is exhibited by a sudden change over a few hours or days in Mom's memory and abilities.

Many families realize there is a dementia problem when memory loss in a parent or spouse becomes increasingly apparent and is at a point where it can no longer be ignored.

But contrary to popular belief, confusion and memory loss are not normal aging. Brain function does not decline with age. Instead, mature adults' thought processes and memories become more advanced and developed as we age. Dementia is a disease of the brain, it is unusual and not the result of normal aging.

Some families report first noticing Mom is having trouble with her finances, or she is having word-finding problems or she is asking the same questions repeatedly, yet she can still maintain a social conversation. Others realize there is a problem because Mom is layering clothing or because Mom's normally neat and tidy house now looks disorganized or smells unclean.

Chapter 1 – Defining Dementia

Still other families suddenly realize that for the past several years, Mom has been slowly losing her abilities and she is having a harder time surviving and performing the daily activities of living (ADLs). ADLs are the things we do every day, such as sleeping, ambulating, toileting, dressing, bathing, grooming or eating.

There are an estimated four dozen dementias. While Alzheimer's is the most common, there is also Multi-Infarct Dementia (previously known as Vascular Dementia), Parkinson's disease, Pick's Disease, Frontotemporal Dementia, Lewy Body Dementia, Substance-Induced Dementia (caused by alcohol abuse or drug abuse), Huntington's disease, Creutzfeldt - Jakob disease, Dementia Due to HIV Disease and Dementia Due to Other General Medical Conditions.

There are some other dementias you may hear about, the so-called "reversible" dementias like normal pressure hydrocephalus or Thyroid-imbalanced dementia, but these dementias are not really "reversible." In reality, the cause of further damage to the brain may be stopped through diagnosis and treatment, but dementia and its cognitive impairment has already been done, i.e., the brain is now damaged. Calling these types of dementia "reversible" leads to further confusion by the public about dementias.

Chapter 1 – Defining Dementia

To better explain the disease processes of dementia, this book is organized into chapters covering the disease history, the Four A's of Dementia, physiological changes, perceptional changes, sensory changes, communication strategies, depression issues, the Global Deterioration Scale's characteristics for the seven stages or levels of dementia, nutrition, activities of daily living – including bathing issues and dressing, grief issues for families and patients, and death.

I wrote this book to explain to families what dementia does to a person physically and emotionally. In over a decade of working as a geriatric social worker and then a gerontologist, I have yet to meet a family who understood what Alzheimer's disease or dementia is, what it will do to the person they love and what will be the end result of the disease.

Most people I meet have simply been told that a person they love has dementia and will have memory problems. With that meager bit of information, they are frequently overwhelmed by the physical and emotional changes that accompany dementia.

This book will explain to families what is going to happen to their loved one physiologically as a result of the disease, what the stages of the disease are, and hopefully

Chapter 1 – Defining Dementia

allow them to understand the disease process in a way that will help them to prepare for the years ahead.

Amazingly enough, too many times the diagnosis of dementia is made in an emergency room while a person was ill with an infection or pneumonia. No actual testing was done by a neurologist or a geriatrician or a geriatric psychiatrist to arrive at the diagnosis of dementia.

No specific type of dementia is assigned to the person and no actual testing for dementia was done other than an emergency room doctor asking an older and very ill person orientation questions such as: "What is your name?" or "Where are you?" or "What is today's date?" and "What is the year?"

Sadly, the result of this can be diagnosing a person with dementia, when she may actually have delirium. To make a more positive diagnosis, your loved one should be examined by a neurologist, a geriatrician (a physician who specializes in adults – the opposite of a pediatrician) or a geriatric psychiatrist. There is a battery of tests to be performed to make a true diagnosis, not simply a standardized set of orientation questions. The result of the testing is a diagnosis made with 95 percent accuracy.

It will be helpful as you seek treatment and information for your parent or spouse that you locate and use a

Chapter 1 – Defining Dementia

geriatrician. After all, you probably took your children to a pediatrician because that doctor specialized in the treatment of children and adolescents; older adults deserve the same kind of specialization for their medical care.

The diagnosis of dementia often leaves a family totally unprepared for the vast physical and emotional changes that will occur to the person they love. Dementia is not just a memory problem; it is a total loss of a person's abilities, talents, personality, physical, mental and emotional traits; the very complex behaviors that make each person unique.

It is devastating to both the families and the person with the dementia. Families can frequently become quite angry and emotional as the disease progresses and they realize what is reality is much different than being told "Your mother has dementia, she's going to lose her memory."

The day to day losses that dementia causes and the end result of the diseases are difficult for families, to say the least. The person you know and love will no longer exist in the way you knew and loved her. As the disease progresses, she will even develop a distinct look inherent to the disease process. In time, she will have a total loss

Chapter 1 – Defining Dementia

of the personality that makes her the person you know. As such, the grieving process families go through, seemingly again and again, is extremely taxing, to say the least.

Dementia is the disease which robs a person of memory and personality, the things which make us who we are. For some families, the disease becomes too difficult to handle and the behaviors exhibited by their loved ones are taken personally, rather than as a process of the disease.

Sons and daughters and spouses may be unable to deal with the emotions of watching a loved one slip away bit by bit, a harrowing process in grief known as "The Long Goodbye."

As the brain shrinks from three pounds to one pound during the course of the disease, the impact on the body system's functions are dramatic and non-reversible, and the brain's ability to interpret and react to the signals and messages is equally impaired.

I believe if families can understand what the disease does to their loved one's brain and how that same brain contains the individual's memories and personality, they will have a better understanding of the resulting behaviors exhibited by their loved one.

Chapter 1 – Defining Dementia

Understanding that behaviors are being driven by a damaged brain, means families will be better prepared to separate the results of their loved one's behaviors from their own emotions.

Unlike some other diseases, dementia does not go into "remission." The various diseases of dementia are aggressive and continue to attack the brain until the person is dead, either from the disease itself or from the failure of another of the body's systems, i.e. the heart or kidneys.

For example, a person with Multi-Infarct Dementia may die from a heart attack or other cardiac event before the cumulative effect of multiple strokes destroys the brain.

Remember there is a common misconception that various organ and systems of the body function independently of one another. The perception is at birth the doctor smacks the baby's bottom; the baby cries and then all the body's systems are functioning independently of each other or in harmony with each other.

And while the doctor may indeed smack the baby's bottom, in reality, the brain controls the body, its systems and its organs.

In actuality, blood circulation, breathing, swallowing, kidney function, respiration, etc., are all ultimately

Chapter 1 – Defining Dementia

controlled by the brain. And because the brain controls all the systems of the body, every system is eventually affected as the brain becomes more and more damaged.

Body temperature, vision, digestion, auditory input and translation, language, heart, circulation, lungs, kidneys, skin, etc.; every system of the body is impaired and affected by the disease. The effects of the disease are seen specifically as each lobe of the brain responsible for each particular function is damaged or destroyed.

So the brain controls organ functioning and interprets for the body incoming signals. These signals include our perceptions of our surroundings. Meaning the brain interrupts what the eyes see, what the mouth tastes, what the ears hear, what the skin feels. from not only the organs, but also what the eyes are seeing, what food tastes like, how sound and noise are interpreted by the ears and what the body is feeling – cold, heat, pain.

Therefore, not only does a loss of ability by the organs to function in their designed capacity occur, but there is also a loss of an ability to see clearly, to hear accurately, to taste food, to perceive pain or temperature, to coordinate muscle movement or to be able to walk; because the brain cannot interpret the signals it is receiving from the senses and respond accordingly.

Chapter 1 – Defining Dementia

Once a specific ability is lost, it cannot be regained or relearned because the brain is too impaired. The part of the brain that controlled that function or ability is damaged and finally destroyed. This is not a use it or lose it scenario, this is a once it's lost, it is gone scenario.

So as the disease progresses, the person is not facing a "use it or lose it" concept. Instead it is a total "lost" concept and no amount or physical therapy or cueing and coaching can bring that ability back. Remember Alzheimer's disease does not stop. It causes damage every moment of every day and with the cumulative effect of the disease, the person you love will change more and more, until she is simply a reminder of the person she once was.

Think of it this way: the brain is the hard drive, the central processor. All of a person's abilities, personality traits and memories are files stored on that hard drive. As the disease progress, files have more and more parts deleted or erased, until the entire file is destroyed. Once a file is gone, it is gone.

Meaning, once your mom loses the ability to walk, she has lost the ability to walk. No amount of physical therapy will change that process. The parts of the brain containing the files for walking are gone and there are no other

Chapter 1 – Defining Dementia

walking files in reserve to draw on. These losses are complete and devastating, to the person and to the family.

One of the difficult aspects of this disease is that Mom doesn't lose her abilities all at once, but little by little. One moment she may not know how to walk, but 30 minutes later she may remember how to walk again. But once her ability to walk is totally gone, it's gone.

It is important to remember at times you may become frustrated because it may appear as though your loved one is "pretending" to not know how to do a task. People with dementia don't have the ability to "pretend" anything. Their brain is under assault by an aggressive disease process. Pretending is not something they are capable of doing. The inability to remember is frustrating and devastating to watch, but actions and recall are not deliberate or planned.

A more positive approach involves looking at the abilities that are left and focusing an individual's goals on realistic targets. If Mom loved baking Christmas cookies or coloring Easter eggs, then make certain she is still a part of that tradition. Even when she can no longer make the cookies, she may be able to decorate.

Chapter 1 – Defining Dementia

When she can no longer decorate, she can still talk about memories and stories of the cookies and past Christmas parties.

As the disease progresses, she can be part of the cooking process and listen as you explain your love for the same activity and your memories of her baking the holiday cookies when you were a child. For example, in the beginning, she can bake cookies without assistance. Then she needs help turning on the oven and gathering the ingredients.

Eventually, she needs help measuring the flour, etc., and in time she can only stir the mixture and talk about her cookies. Finally, in the final stages, she will be able to enjoy her time with you and smell the old memories of baking the cookies, long after her abilities to actively participate are gone.

The goals of the activities change as Mom loses more of her abilities, but the activity continues with more and more input from you and others close to her.

This book will also discuss in detail the Global Deterioration Score and Scale. This is a tool used to determine which stage of the disease your loved one is in. The behaviors exhibited by a person determine the stage of the disease. Regardless of which dementia a person

Chapter 1 – Defining Dementia

has, all of the dementias can be graded on the GDS, based on the behavior characteristics exhibited by a person. These stages or levels allow professionals and families to determine where in the disease process a person falls and thus gives you a measurement of time to prepare for the future of the disease process.

The Global Deterioration Scale and its behaviors will be discussed in detail in Chapter Seven.

For many of you, this book will be the first time this information will be presented. It may be difficult to read as you may find the information or scenarios are too familiar to your family and loved one. If that should happen, set the book aside and come back to it later.

Remember this information is being presented in a straight forward and clinical manner, but the reality of the disease for you may be altogether different, because the disease is affecting our loved one or someone you love.

2

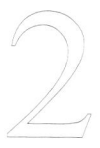

History of Dementia

For thousands of years, a disease process we call dementia has been described in Western literature. Indeed, even the earliest writings of medicine describe behaviors, illnesses and death which could only be caused by one of the dementias. Believe it or not, you already know this.

Think about kings and emperors who went "mad" or references to people who had "shaky disease." They are easy to find in history and literature. In my own lifetime, I would hear of an older person who was confused and "senile" or had developed "hardening of the arteries." We now recognize these disease processes as forms of dementia. But the more formal "discovery" of the Alzheimer's disease process began only a few hundred years ago. In the book, *How We Die*, Dr. Sherwin B. Nuland describes the discovery of Alzheimer's disease.

Chapter 2 – History of Dementia

French physician Philippe Pinel, in 1801, coined the term "demence" to mean an "incoherence" of the mental faculties. Pinel was describing an unusual disease process in a 34-year-old woman he was treating.

Over the course of three years, the young woman lost her memory (amnesia), the ability to speak (aphasia), the ability to recognize objects or people (agnosia) and the ability to walk, eat or swallow (apraxia.) (These are the "Four A's of Alzheimer's" discussed in Chapter Three.)

One of Pinel's students, Dr. Jean Esquirol, treated a female patient with similar behaviors in 1838. Following her autopsy, Esquirol documented the damage and changes he saw in the woman's brain.

"Convolutions of the brain are atrophied, separated from one another or flattened, compressed and small, especially in the frontal regions," he wrote. Pinel had also described areas of his patient's brain as "depressed, atrophied, and almost destroyed, and the empty space filled with serum."

In 1907, a 39-year-old German physician published a paper entitled *"On a Distinctive Disease of the Cerebral Cortex."* He reported his study of a 51-year-old female who had been hospitalized in a psychiatric hospital in 1901 and had gone through a succession of symptoms

Chapter 2 – History of Dementia

before death. They included "jealousy, failure of memory, paranoia, loss of reasoning powers, incomprehension, stupor" and death after four and one-half years.

This particular doctor had developed great skill in the newly developed area of tissue-staining techniques. He was already known as the doctor who first identified the changes in cellular structure specific to syphilis, Huntington's chorea, arteriosclerosis and senility.

But when he autopsied the woman's brain and studied the stained tissue under a microscope, Alois Alzheimer made the discovery for which he is remembered. Using an optical microscope, Alzheimer determined from the autopsy of the woman that she had brain cells that had disappeared altogether or contained dense bundles of fibrils where the nucleus and the brain cell should have been.

Between one-fourth and one-third of the brain showed these structural changes. The brain had also atrophied and filled with cerebrospinal fluid, as had been previously documented by Pinel and others, but there were also bone-like structures located around the nerve endings. The end result of the damage was a one pound brain.

Alzheimer's conclusion became a universal understatement. "We are apparently confronted with a

Chapter 2 – History of Dementia

distinctive disease process," he wrote. When Alzheimer's mentor Dr. Emil Kraepelin wrote his eighth medical textbook in 1910, he referred to this "new" entity as Alzheimer's disease.

So, a diagnosis of Alzheimer's means that there are four distinct physiological events (See Chapter Five) occurring in the brain. First, the sulci or outer creases of the brain, which normally lay tightly folded against each other as the brain is snuggled in the cranium, are opening up as the brain shrivels.

At the end of the disease, the shrinking has caused these folds to shrivel up and in doing so, open to a point where you could place your finger or a pencil in between the grooves in space that didn't exist before.

Secondly, in the center part of the brain, the temporal lobe normally has a small bit of cerebrospinal fluid in it. By the end stages of Alzheimer's, the Temporal Lobe and the Frontal Lobe will be full of cerebrospinal fluid. The Temporal Lobe controls language, hearing and smell. The Frontal Lobe controls personality, memory, attention, cognition, rational thought, memory and judgment.

As these areas are destroyed, you can better understand why your loved one is changing; after all, look at all the things these two lobes control.

Chapter 2 – History of Dementia

Thirdly, the nucleus in individual brain cells is coming apart. No longer neat and functional, the nucleus is now coming apart inside its cell. There are dense bundles of fibrils, neurofibillary tangles and a buildup of protein clumps. The once neat nucleus now resembles a plate of spaghetti in structure.

Fourth, the "housekeeping" cells in the brain have turned off. Dead nerve cells are no longer being carried from the brain. Instead the dead cells begin to build up around the endings of the nerves. The result is plaque, but not a soft pulpy plaque. This is a bony-like structure that feels like sand or grit and it's now growing in the soft tissue of the brain.

The final result of these four changes is devastating to the person and her family. A healthy adult brain that weighed three pounds and had 100 billion brain cells, a brain that was normal and allowed your loved one to be the person she was, now weighs only about one pound. The remaining five billion or so brain cells are heavily damaged and have great difficulty sustaining life.

The person you love is struggling every day during this disease process to make sense of a world that is becoming more and more confusing and to understand stimuli that no longer have meaning as the disease

Chapter 2 – History of Dementia

continues its attack. Changes seem to occur more rapidly towards the end of the disease process, because of the cumulative effect of the disease. Losing a few hundred thousand or even million brain cells in the beginning doesn't have too much effect, because there are so many healthy brain cells still functioning. But over time, the effects are easily noticeable when you are observing her speech and behavior.

Towards the final stages, the changes are detectable in her every movement, her facial features and every component of her daily life.

It is perhaps a strange twist of fate that this doctor's name was Alzheimer. In my native Texas, our slow drawl leads to a pronunciation which transforms the word into "Old Timer's Disease." Those two little words, "old timer's," further advances the fallacy that dementia is a normal part of aging, when it is in reality, the opposite and not normal aging.

Most people live at home until their final few days and most elderly people learn at the age of 80 at the same rate they learned at the age of 20. Older folks may be a little slower on testing as they are out of practice, but given enough time, their learning skills and cognition are intact.

Chapter 2 – History of Dementia

At present there are an estimated 5.7 million Americans with Alzheimer's disease. As the 77 million member Baby Boomer population ages, that number is expected to increase to between 17 and 20 million Americans.

These figures do not mean a greater number of people are "catching" Alzheimer's; it simply represents a huge population group moving through the aging process. There are more Baby Boomers; hence there are more people with Alzheimer. And since Alzheimer's accounts for sixty to eighty of all dementia cases, that means five to 10 million other types of dementia are also attacking Americans.

The exact figure for the number of people with a dementia is difficult to ascertain as people can suffer more than one dementia at a time, a condition known as dual dementia.

A decade ago, estimates for the cost of care for Americans with Alzheimer's was more than $40 billion annually. The cost for the Baby Boomer population will start at a staggering $500 billion dollars and is expected to reach into the trillions of dollars. That is more than the Federal Government's current entire budget for Medicaid and Medicare.

Chapter 2 – History of Dementia

It is no small wonder then that all assisted living and skilled nursing facilities market an Alzheimer's specific program. The business process of caring for the elderly is attempting to capture an exploding Baby Boomer market, but sadly, the owners are not educated on the disease process.

They market Alzheimer's care as more expensive and occurring in a controlled and locked environment, but have no real knowledge or concept of the entire disease process. Many companies actually have programs and policies in place which are detrimental to the aging process of Alzheimer's.

For example, some programs use colored plates at mealtimes, and market those colored plates as a "signature" of their business. But the color of the plate can actually stop a dementia resident from eating or even seeing the food. Some programs are using activity items designed for persons who are recovering from a brain-injury or designed to stimulate a mentally retarded brain. The effect of these items is that they cause greater confusion for the demented person and tend to increase that person's paranoia and combative behavior.

Any properly designed and implemented program should feature structured and stage appropriate activities,

Chapter 2 – History of Dementia

that is, activities designed for the specific stage of the disease process your loved one is currently in. The staff should be able to assess for those stages and be able to explain the stages to families. That same staff should be constantly undergoing training and role-playing to ensure consistency and understanding of the disease process.

Meals and types of food should be planned and designed with advanced dementia stages in mind. Snacks should be sweet to appeal to the loss of taste and high calorie to offset the calorie burning effects of the disease. Alcohol and caffeine should not be served due to the detrimental effect on a person with dementia.

The persons in charge of dementia programs also need specialized training. Some companies will only hire persons for their dementia programs who have formalized knowledge or training in aging, i.e. a bachelor's or masters in gerontology, social work, psychology or nursing.

Other companies have a history of promoting care givers who exhibit some leadership skills. Unfortunately, dementia programs need directors trained and educated in the process of aging, not simply a person who is kind to the elderly and loyal to the company. This is a serious disease. If someone you love has Alzheimer's or another

Chapter 2 – History of Dementia

of the dementias, you are facing a great challenge and years of heartache. The dementia patient deserves the best care we can offer.

The logic of placing a non-educated person in charge of a dementia facility escapes me. It is akin to saying because I can put a Band-Aid over a scraped knee, I should be in charge of an emergency room. You would never allow that nor would you visit my emergency room for care or treatment.

Dementia requires professionals to design and implement programs to care for the people with Alzheimer's, not persons who don't know or understand the differences between the diseases of dementia.

We know enough about the disease process now to have better designed and consistent programming, the challenge for families is insisting those programs be made available. If the companies understand they will not get the thousands of dollars they demand monthly without it, then change and real, professional care giving will occur.

3

The Four A's of Dementia

As a family deals with this dementia, there are four medical terms describing the effects of the disease on the person. Your doctor or health professional may use these terms, often referred to as "The Four A's of Alzheimer's disease." The Four A's are amnesia, agnosia, aphasia and apraxia. The "Four A's" are exhibited in all the dementias.

These "Four A's" are represented individually in behaviors or in conjunction with each other in behavior as their specific components overlap at times. For example, both amnesia and agnosia lead to confusion about people's identity, but for different reasons.

When family members observe amnesia, apraxia, agnosia or aphasia in their loved one, they are witnessing the very behaviors that allow for the placement of their loved one on the Global Deterioration Scale. It is

Chapter 3 - The Four A's of Dementia

important to understand it is the disease or specific dementia causing the behaviors, actions and reactions witnessed by the family.

Understanding that these behaviors are a part of the disease process helps us to not take words, actions or events personally or feel attacked when the behavior is directed specifically at us. Observing these behaviors allows families to help professionals grade where the dementia patient is medically and gather more information to determine the stage represented at that time.

Remember, there is meaning in all behavior. In other words, behavior in people with dementia means something, it is a clue to what that person is feeling or needing. You will find that the very behaviors you have witnessed in your mom are actually common to the disease process; many times those strange, confusing behaviors are actually hallmark features of the disease.

When you are being accused of stealing, or of being another person, when you are listening to repeated sentences, words, stories or questions; you are witnessing a normal part of the disease process. And these are just some of the behaviors you may be constantly confronted with from your loved one.

Chapter 3 - The Four A's of Dementia

The "Four A's" help us understand where those behaviors are originating and why there is a logic to them. I can promise you every family sees these same behaviors, and the behaviors are simply clues to what the disease is doing to the brain.

Knowing and understanding these medical terms will also prove helpful when you are discussing the disease process with your loved one's physician. Describing these behaviors will assist your doctor in prescribing the proper medications to hopefully allow Mom to maintain a higher level of control and abilities for a longer time.

Learning these terms and what they represent should also allow family members to keep a clearer perspective as the disease progresses and remember the disease is responsible for behaviors that are upsetting or out of character, rather than the person.

Amnesia

Amnesia is typically the first sign the family sees in their loved one indicating there is a cognitive problem. This is not the amnesia of television soap operas, but rather a true amnesia where the affected person does not remember recent conversations, and will continuously repeat questions or stories. This behavior can be very

Chapter 3 - The Four A's of Dementia

stressful to family members who do not understand why a normally organized mother continues to ask the same questions over and over.

A person's personality, memory, attention, cognition, rational thought, judgment, and imagination are found in the frontal lobes. As the dementia progresses, the individual cells in that area of the brain are disappearing, the neurons in the cells that are left are disrupted and the entire lobe is slowly filling with cerebrospinal fluid.

Amnesia commonly leads to accusations directed towards the family or care givers; "Why didn't you give me breakfast this morning?" "Where did you put my hand bag?" "You stole my purse!" "You stole my car!"

Because of amnesia, the person with Alzheimer's cannot remember where she placed her purse. Imagine how you would respond to the same situation. You come home from work every day and put your purse or keys or briefcase in the same place.

If suddenly that purse was gone and you couldn't find it, you would naturally suspect the other person in the house and ask where your purse is. You might even become worried or frantic and demand to know where your purse is. Because you know you are a responsible

Chapter 3 - The Four A's of Dementia

person and you keep up with your stuff and when things are missing it is only logical to you that the other person took them.

Later when you find that purse in the freezer you are now certain the other person in your house is not only a thief, but also a mean and sneaky person. After all, why would you have put your purse in the freezer? Only a mean or crazy person would do that. And you know you are not mean or crazy, so it must be the other person in the house stealing and hiding your purse.

Amnesia can also cause the Alzheimer's person to become upset when he or she can no longer identify a spouse. Imagine how frightened you would be to wake up next to a total stranger. Families report one parent attacking the other parent because amnesia causes the first parent to be unable to recognize or remember the second parent.

It is common to hear reports from families that their father threatened to call the police when he woke up next to their mother, the woman he has been married to for decades. After all, their father did not want his wife to come home and find this "other woman" in their house,

Chapter 3 - The Four A's of Dementia

especially when he doesn't recognize her and he knows he would not bring another woman home with him.

This process of amnesia may cause individual to repeat questions or stories continually, which can cause family care givers to lose patience and become frustrated with the patient. The care giver often reports feeling guilty later for "snapping" and for becoming angry.

Amnesia also causes the affected individual to wonder, "Am I in the right place, am I doing the right thing?" The world which has always had order for her and has made sense is now a confusing and scary place to be.

Try to imagine if, in this moment, you weren't really certain what your name was or where you were or what you were supposed to be doing. Imagine trying to remember if the chair you are sitting in is in your house. Look around your house, is this really where you live, are these really your things, who are the photographs of the people in the picture frames?

There is a strange sense of familiarity, but then again there is a great deal of confusion jumbled in the mix. The world is becoming a frightening place and your home, where most of us feel safest, no longer feels like home and no longer feels safe. Your loved one may begin to

Chapter 3 - The Four A's of Dementia

insist this is not her home and demand to be returned to her mother's house, because that is what she remembers as home.

Think of memory as a building block process. First you learned "Mama" and "Daddy" and then you learned "Please" and "Thank you." Then everything began to build on top of that first knowledge. This means that social skills remain strong to the end of life; therefore, if I am polite, the person with Alzheimer's is polite back to me. But it also means memories are being lost in a reverse order of how memories were formed.

In other words, most recent events are lost first or are not able to be learned at all. A person will forget her last born child first and remember her first born child longest. This is due to there being more memories imbedded of that first born child. Eventually she will forget her children and then her husband and so how could she remember children if she cannot remember being married?

As she does not remember being married or having children, she will fall back onto long term memory, such as childhood or young adulthood memories of her mother and father and siblings. So when she now thinks of home, that childhood home is where she knows she needs to go.

Chapter 3 - The Four A's of Dementia

But her children may resemble someone she does remember, such as a father or mother or sister or brother, cousin, aunt or uncle, so she will refer to her child as that person.

But amnesia can also mean she remembers who each child is, but cannot remember the correct word to describe that child. So she may introduce her son as her husband or her daughter as her mother.

This amnesia occurs earlier in the disease process and is considered to be a confusion of words, rather than memory. She is pulling words to describe family members from the pool of family words, but just getting the wrong word.

Likewise she may use words from other pools of words to explain feelings or wants or needs. For example, she may talk about water or rain or wetness, but she is not describing the weather. Rather she is talking about needing to go to the bathroom or needing a drink of water.

Amnesia also means a person is forgetting how to do specific tasks. She can no longer remember how to add or subtract numbers correctly. Many family members begin to first realize there is a serious problem because they find bills unpaid or hidden away because Mom no longer

Chapter 3 - The Four A's of Dementia

knows what to do with the bills. She may pay the electric bill several times in one month or may not pay it at all. She may be giving vast amounts of money to family members or strangers without fully realizing what she is doing.

Amnesia means she can no longer remember how to cook food properly, work a stove correctly or remember how to drive. She may not remember eating and may insist she be fed again, or insist she doesn't need any food because she thinks she has already eaten.

Amnesia is why we don't correct Mom, but rather go along with her perceptions and memories. Her reality is your reality. If she believes it is 1975 and she still has a husband and she is looking for him, we never tell her the reality, which is that her husband died several years ago. Instead, we tell her a logical place her husband would be: at work, at the golf course or bowling alley, etc.

Trying to correct amnesia creates greater confusion and paranoia for your loved one and leads that person to have possible outbursts or aggression as Mom becomes convinced you are lying to her. Always, her reality is your reality.

Chapter 3 - The Four A's of Dementia

Imagine how you felt the day you received devastating news about the loss of a loved one. Perhaps it was the telephone call telling you your other parent had died or your spouse had been killed in an accident. To constantly correct your loved one about the status of the person she is missing and looking for is cruel and forces her to relive that moment of grief time and again. Where she is right now is just that, it's where she is. Her reality is your reality. In the final stage of the disease, amnesia is complete and the person no longer knows herself.. This is a long and difficult progression to this final point.

Agnosia

Agnosia is the second "A" of Alzheimer's and is the inability to recognize common objects or people. Reread that sentence. It says common objects or people. That means your mom is not just confusing a fork with a spoon, or a toothbrush with a hairbrush, it means she is beginning to confuse people she should know, calling them by the wrong name, referring to a son as a husband, a daughter as a mother or an aunt or a sister. In the final stages, she may not recognize people as people.

Agnosia is also the part of the disease process exhibited when mom placed her purse in the refrigerator

Chapter 3 - The Four A's of Dementia

and accused you of stealing it and putting it there to hide it from her. It means she didn't recognize the purse as a purse in that moment nor did she recognize the refrigerator as the wrong place to store her purse.

But it also means the disease process in which she will eventually no longer recognize people as people has begun. Again imagine as you go through your day not being certain who or what the other people you encounter are. How frightening is the world and our environment when we no longer know who people are or what people are?

Agnosia causes the individual to become lost in what should be a familiar place. For example, the individual does not recognize the bathroom or know what to do once in the bathroom. As the disease progresses, the person will no longer receive and understand a signal from the brain that her bladder or bowel is full, and incontinence will begin.

The person may experience anxiety because she does not recognize food items, utensils, common appliances or her own home. The individual may also not recognize family members and may order them out of the house. She may accuse her spouse of being an imposter and

Chapter 3 - The Four A's of Dementia

threaten to call the police or become combative to protect herself from this "stranger."

Think of how you would react if suddenly strangers appeared in your house. You would be frightened, possibly aggressive and threatening. Many people become angry when they feel threatened and dementia patients are no different. You would want the police to assist you and you might scream out for help.

This part of agnosia can be embarrassing for families. Your loved one may call 911 repeatedly because she is trying to call you, but can only remember the shorter number. She may call you repeatedly in the middle of the night because she no longer recognizes time or day and night.

She may frantically insist you come to her and she may describe in detail assaults or attacks from others. She is no longer able to make sense out of common objects or people. She now suffers from delusions and hallucinations as she can't make sense of her world.

Amnesia and agnosia overlap each other and lead to further confusion and behaviors. Here's an example: Lorraine was a clothing buyer for a large company. She

Chapter 3 - The Four A's of Dementia

was always extremely well-dressed. She came up to me and said she was missing "Something."

I could tell she was discussing clothing, but didn't know if it was pants or a blouse, so I pointed and touched my clothing and hers. It was pants.

"Okay," I said, "Are you missing the silk pants or the cotton pants?" I asked the name of every fabric I knew trying to figure out what pants we were looking for. The answer was always a frustrated "No!"

Finally, Lorraine blurted out "The Army pants, my Army pants."

Now to work with dementia, it is helpful and recommended you know and understand history for that generation of people. "Army pants" to a person who lived through World War II and whose husband was a career officer can only be one thing.

"We are looking for your khaki pants, right Lorraine?"

She began to cry with relief. "Yes, yes, yes!"

Not being able to say "khaki" or "pants" in the beginning was agnosia and amnesia and aphasia all rolled into one. Dementia frequently requires you to be both a detective

Chapter 3 - The Four A's of Dementia

and a behavioralist as you try to make sense out of the clues you are given.

In the final stage, agnosia is complete and the person won't know how to use any item or recognize people.

Aphasia

Aphasia is the third "A" of Alzheimer's disease. It is the inability to either use or understand language. This disease process can cause the individual to provide a lengthy description of an item when she cannot find word. She may replace one word with another word, leading to confusing speech.

Aphasia overlaps with amnesia and agnosia in word finding processes and indicates the Temporal Lobe is being attacked and damaged. (Lorraine was also exhibiting aphasia when she couldn't remember the name of the pants she was missing.)

Sometimes the inserted word is an unrelated word. Sometimes it is a word from the same pool of words, i.e. terms for different family members, referring to a son as "my husband." She may talk about water or rain or a bath and be asking for a drink or water or the bathroom.

Chapter 3 - The Four A's of Dementia

Aphasia often leads to increased anxiety in families when the individual calls a family member by the wrong name or refers to his wife as his mother. He may actually know exactly who the individual is, but may just be experiencing difficulty with word-finding, usually in the earlier stages of the disease process. Or as the disease advances, he may truly have confused the two individuals.

Aphasia and the other A's mean using all your skills to understand what your loved one is saying.

You may find you are actually quite adept at reading behavior. Most of our communication with each other does not involve words. Instead, it involves reading someone's body language, her movement, her facial reactions, etc. We are really very good at understanding what people around us are communicating or trying to communicate; it's just that sometimes we forget. Remember, this ability will prove invaluable when the ability to speak is lost.

Think about communication this way. You probably have children. I doubt any of you brought your baby home from the hospital and that child was walking or talking. Yet you could tell when that baby was hungry or needed changing or was ill, sad or happy. You did all of that

Chapter 3 - The Four A's of Dementia

without the baby being able to speak. With your parent or spouse, you will use those same skills again and again to determine what is needed or what hurts.

Aphasia, agnosia and amnesia processes all overlap and add to the increased confusion of the person.

In the final stage, the person will be unable to use or understand any language.

Apraxia

Apraxia is the fourth "A" of Alzheimer's. It is the inability of the brain to coordinate purposeful movement. Simply put, Alzheimer's patients fall down because the brain is too damaged to be able to tell the body how to stay in balance while standing, preparing to stand or sit or walk. The brain is now becoming too damaged to tell the body how to swallow food correctly or to use a fork or a toothbrush or allow a person to dress or undress.

Alzheimer's disease eventually causes problems with balance or movements as the brain shrinks and deteriorates and is no longer able to signal the muscular structure for movement.

In the final stage, the person can no longer sit up or hold her head up correctly, she will no longer be able to

Chapter 3 - The Four A's of Dementia

chew or swallow food. She will be incontinent. She will require total care and supervision.

In addition to the loss of muscle movement and coordination, the Occipital Lobe of the brain is deteriorating and the person no longer sees the environment with depth-perception, but the brain interprets the world around her as flat, much the way a photograph appears.

The individual may reach for something on the table and miss the item. The individual may have difficulty catching a ball or clapping his hands. Sometimes, those with Alzheimer's disease describe situations where the floor feels as though it is moving. Some are very fearful of steps because the steps seem to be in motion.

Between the damage to the Occipital Lobe and the onset of apraxia, your loved one is at great risk to walk into desks, chairs, doorways, etc., because coordination and depth perception is damaged.

As apraxia advances, the gait becomes affected. The step itself becomes shuffling and shorter, which increases the risk for falling. The foot isn't completely lifted before each step, increasing the risk of falling or stumbling. And because of dementia, the person doesn't realize the risk and can become combative when you attempt to assist.

Your mom may pick up a glass of juice and be unable to get it to her mouth. She may pour it on the table or drop it. She may pour it into her plate of food because she became confused between picking up the juice to drink and getting it to her mouth. Or she may have forgotten what to do with the glass once she picked it up.

Apraxia affects all muscular movement, including smiling. As apraxia advances, the facial features become flatter with little affect, another hallmark feature of the disease.

In the final stage, a person will be unable to walk, sit up, hold her head up, chew or swallow. She will have a complete loss of ability to utilize her muscular structure.

4

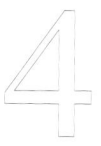

Physiological Changes

The vast cellular and structural changes occurring in the brains of people with Alzheimer's mean the affected persons have a tremendous challenge making sense of the world around them. During normal aging, the body's organ systems begin to decline in function very slowly.

This decrease begins once the adult passes the age of 35. Some systems lose ability at one per cent of functioning per year. Remember these changes are slow and gradual and the body makes adjustments throughout life to compensate for this.

But even within this normal aging process, dementia is just not normal. The brain has some structural changes related to aging, but a lifetime of living experiences brings about rich dendritic and neuron growth. The normally aging brain of a mature elderly person is actually quite powerful and complex and not at all the stereotyped

Chapter 4 - Psychological Changes

befuddled and confused elderly person portrayed on television.

Common changes during normal aging also include a gradually stooped posture and possible weight loss. The body's skin has a diminished ability to sweat, and is wrinkled and drier. The eyes have some loss of peripheral vision, a decreased sensitivity to color (hence a favorite color can be red, because it can be seen more easily), some loss of visual clarity and depth perception, and a decreased adaptation to light changes.

There is some hearing loss, as the inner ear's moveable pieces become stiffer and vibrate less readily, and the cochlea ages. The mouth has a decreased taste perception and a harder time salivating. The lungs have a decreased reserve capacity and the skeleton suffers a loss of bone tissue and painful arthritic changes in the joints.

For women who have given birth, the loss of calcium makes for fragile bones. Often these women can suffer a hip fracture while standing and then fall rather than falling and having the hip break because of contact with the floor.

There is a lessened ability of the heart to respond to stress and a lower pulse rate in normal aging. Mobility is

Chapter 4 - Psychological Changes

affected by a lessened ability to move quickly. The kidneys have an increased frequency of urination. The central nervous system shows a decrease in the hours of sleep received, and there is a decrease in the sense of smell, sensitivity to hot or cold and the older adult has slower reflexes.

But the brain, even with some slight structural changes remains fully functional. Changes in brain function that occur with aging are more than likely related to the fact that people are no longer using their brains as they did when they were younger.

For example, an 80-year-old person is typically retired, does not read as much as before, is somewhat structured in her everyday life and simply does not challenge her brain the same way a college student or young adult does. Remember her brain is richer in dendritic growth and neurons, due to a lifetime of experiences.

It is much more complex than that of a 20-year-old person. And given enough time to take a test, she will do just as well as she did in her younger years. Again, dementia is not normal aging.

But even with all of these changes, in normal aging, the body's various systems are still quite functional into the 10th decade of life (90 years). In a person with

Chapter 4 - Psychological Changes

Alzheimer's, the various organ systems of the body remain in similarly good working order, but the brain can no longer send or receive signals from those organs for correct functioning, due to the daily cumulative damage being inflicted upon the brain.

The end result is that the body's systems begin to operate less efficiently. The changes to the brain affect all organ systems by the final stage, because the damaged brain can no longer signal the body how to operate.

Changes in the Alzheimer Brain

There are four distinct features of a dementia brain, especially an Alzheimer's brain. These distinctions were first documented by Dr. Pinel, Dr. Esquirol and then Dr. Alzheimer with his powerful optical microscope, as discussed in Chapter Two.

To start, a healthy human brain weighs three pounds and contains an estimated 100 billion brain cells. But by Level Seven of the Alzheimer's or dementia's disease process, the brain only weighs around one pound and contains approximately five billion brain cells and a vast number of those cells can not function correctly. Then brain literally shrinks and shrivels during the disease process.

Chapter 4 - Psychological Changes

First, the outer folds of the brain, called sulci, which are tight and folded together on a normal brain, have shrunk and pulled away from each other. (These are the characteristic "wrinkles" we see on the outer structure of the brain.) These outer folds of the brain, which before were tightly laid against each other, now have enough space to allow for a finger or a pencil to go between the folds.

This shrinkage, or atrophy of the cerebral gyri, contributes to the major damage in the areas of the brain controlling higher function; such as memory, language, learning and judgment. This shrinkage leads to the brain no longer being tightly contained within the cranium, meaning there will eventually be a half-inch or more of space between the brain and the skull.

Secondly, major areas of the brain begin to fill with cerebrospinal fluid and have enlarged ventricles. The brain's central areas: the Temporal Lobe (language, hearing and smell), the Frontal Lobe (memory, speech, personality, cognition, attention, judgment, imagination and rational thought) become filled with this cerebrospinal fluid. Normally, there is only a tiny area in the central part of the brain that contains cerebrospinal fluid.

Chapter 4 - Psychological Changes

These two lobes, especially the Frontal Lobe, are the driving force in what makes you uniquely you. So as these lobes are destroyed, all the things that make a person distinctly different are damaged or destroyed. This damage, especially to the Frontal Lobe, is what most impacts a person's personality traits, the individualized traits that make you who you are.

Amnesia's effects are driven by this damage because this is the lobe with memory, personality, attention, cognition, rational thought, judgment, speech and imagination

The third area of destruction in the brain occurs through the accumulation of plaque. During the course of Alzheimer's, the "housekeeping" cells in the brain turn off and stop removing dead nerve cells. These dead cells slowly build-up around the nerve endings in the brain, forming plaque.

This plaque is not a soft, pulpy plaque like what would be found in our arteries; rather it is a bone-like structure. If you could feel it, the plaque would feel like sand or grit between your fingers. This plaque wraps around the endings of the brain's nerve cells. So now the soft tissue of the brain actually has bone structures forming in it.

Chapter 4 - Psychological Changes

Finally, neurofibillary tangles form in the individual brain cells. These tangles occur when the nucleus in the brain cell comes apart. Where there was once a normal brain cell with a complete nucleus, there is now a cell structure with a clump of tangled fibers where a nucleus should be.

If you were to view this cell under a microscope, it would resemble something more like a plate of spaghetti than a functioning nucleus. Clumps of protein are also forming and depositing throughout the brain in this process.

This damage to the brain is continuous and aggressive. Dementia does not stop or go into remission. Current medications are thought to slow the process, but those medicines only work for a short period of time and they only work for some people.

In the beginning of the disease process, the effects are not seen as readily. This is because the brain has 100 billion cells and as a few thousand or even million become damaged, the brain is still able to function. The brain can still find undamaged pathways for signals to get through. A thought is still able to be completed, a sentence still makes sense, and movement can still be completed successfully.

Chapter 4 - Psychological Changes

When you see your mom misspeak and unable to complete a thought, but then, just a few moments later, she makes perfect sense, you are witnessing the brain finding an undamaged pathway. But as time goes on and the damage continues, the cumulative effect is devastating. Thoughts can't be completed, sentences can't be finished in a way that makes sense, movement becomes less and less certain and stable.

By Level Six of the disease, the amount of damage being done to the brain on a daily basis is equivalent to a daily concussion. Imagine someone striking the head daily with a baseball bat. The person's brain is struggling daily to function against the continuous onslaught of the disease process.

This is why structure in the day to day life of persons with Alzheimer's is so important. They need to be able to safely navigate in a less complex environment, one that allows them to still make sense of their surroundings, one with controlled noise, appropriate activities and food they can taste and eat.

So as you can now see, the overall damage to the brain during the course of the disease is extraordinary. The brain will finally weigh only about one pound, its cells will collapse, disintegrate, or fill with a mass of tangles,

Chapter 4 - Psychological Changes

fluid will replace entire lobes and clumps of plaque composed of degenerated portions of axons will cluster around cores of beta-amyloid at the nerve endings, plaque will grow.

These are the hallmark medical features of the disease. A true diagnosis of Alzheimer's can only be made through a brain biopsy or an autopsy, but physicians can currently make the diagnosis accurately in 95 percent of cases by observing the patient's behavior and through neurological testing.

Perceptions of Their World

Visual Changes

As the disease progresses, a person with Alzheimer's will gradually lose her ability to clearly see the environment around her. She may bump into doorways, desks, chairs, couches or tables. She may be unable to clearly see the people around her and together with her amnesia; she will be unable to properly identify persons she should know. Her brain cannot interpret what her eye is seeing, causing an even greater state of confusion.

Meaning, it is not the eye itself that is damaged, but the Occipital Lobe in the brain. As with other systems and senses, it is not the organ that is damaged, but the part of the brain that controls or interprets what that particular organ does that is damaged.

Chapter 5 - Perceptions of Their World

The Occipital Lobe is located in the lower back portion of the brain. If you feel the back of your head, it is the knob above your neck. The Occipital Lobe controls visual association, that is, depth and distance perception. As Mom's visual perception changes from three-dimensional to a flatter one-dimensional interpretation, the world around her begins to looks more and more like a photograph. And as she enters Level Six of the disease process, she will lose her peripheral vision as well.

This causes great difficulty for the person to judge distance, the location of one item to the next. Look around you. You probably have no difficulty distinguishing the distance between your chair and the television, or your chair and the wall or the doorway, or your chair and the window. Imagine now how it would be to not be able to tell that there is distance and instead of that distinction in depth, the world around you was flat.

And when Mom loses her peripheral vision, she can no longer see people approaching her on the side. I have had many instances where I was asked to assess a combative person, a person who was swinging out and striking at care givers. When the person was observed, it was frequently a loss of peripheral vision causing the outburst.

Chapter 5 - Perceptions of Their World

Imagine tonight when you are home and walking down the hallway to your kitchen. How would you react if I suddenly jumped out next to you? Would you scream? Would you instinctively swing at me? Would your innate "startle reflex" kick in to protect you from danger or harm? That same reaction for being startled and frightened is what a person with Alzheimer's feels when a person seems to suddenly "jump" out at her.

As a result, always walk around an Alzheimer's person at arm's length when you are approaching her from behind and talk to the person and tell her you are coming around her. Touch her on the shoulder while you are talking to help her gauge where you are and associate your voice with the person suddenly appearing at her side. You are less likely to get hit and she is less likely to be scared.

Remember, with the changes in the brain's ability to understand the environment, if is incumbent upon us to do everything possible to make the world easier to navigate and understand. Imagine how frightened you would feel if being startled and scared by persons suddenly seeming to jump out at you throughout the day was a regular event. The Alzheimer person's world is becoming more and more confusing and scary.

Chapter 5 - Perceptions of Their World

Visual changes mean everything around Mom is affected. A nicely waxed floor, at home, in a skilled nursing facility or hospital, looks shiny, bright and clean to you and me. To a person with Alzheimer's, those waxed floors appear more like water. The step into the elevator is just a step to you and me.

But to Mom, that step seems perilous. It is a step marked by a shiny bar and then a different colored floor. Have you noticed Mom tapping the floor with her foot when she goes from one color or texture to another?

That wonderfully decorated room, with its hardwood floors followed by soft carpet, are seen as possible holes, rather than flooring. This confusion visually is a combination of the symptoms of agnosia, amnesia and apraxia. Imagine when you leave your office and walk to the building's entrance. Is the floor a different color? Now look at the sidewalk. Is it another color as well? And the parking lot or street. What color is asphalt? What color are deep holes? And aren't most parking lots set about six to eight inches below the sidewalk? Have you ever missed the step from the sidewalk to the parking lot or street?

Imagine how that felt and then imagine if every step you were taking felt as though it would result in a misstep, as though at any second, you could fall.

Chapter 5 - Perceptions of Their World

Remember with the way the disease process works, Mom may remember her room location at some point in the day, but she may not remember it later. Bright name signs and other decorations will assist her in finding her room as the decorations help make the door look more distinctive and identifiable.

If your mom is living in a facility like a nursing home or an assisted living building, when she looks down a hallway, it looks long and empty, with no unusual color to break up the view. You and I can still gauge distance and see depth, Mom cannot.

The rooms in facilities generally look alike and regular door markers typically have small numbers and postage stamp sized photos of the residents. Those markers are usually located about 70 inches above the floor. But many residents are in wheelchairs or they are not tall enough to see the identifying numbers for their rooms. Be creative in finding ways to help your mom locate her room. Using the color red is a favorite, because elderly people can see red more clearly than softer colors like blue and green.

People with Alzheimer's can also be overwhelmed by too much visual stimuli. In a normal brain, the brain itself applies a value to the stimuli input it is receiving. When you are driving, for example, your brain focuses on the

Chapter 5 - Perceptions of Their World

cars and movements it needs to focus on. When you are sitting in your office, your brain filters noise and movement it deems unnecessary to allow you to focus on what is important, the task at hand.

But for a diseased and damaged brain, that filtering system is lost. It is incumbent upon the care giver to help the brain filter stimuli. Dining, for example, needs to be a quiet time. When eating, providing a controlled and structured environment is especially important.

Too many distractions can cause a hungry person to not be able to eat because her brain cannot filter out the environment around her and focus on eating. Her brain is overwhelmed and she is simply stopped in the process. Stereos, televisions, loud talking, movement by others, tables decorated with flowers, condiments, multiple glassware and silverware, all these things can be overwhelming to a person with Alzheimer's.

As the disease progresses, keep plates simple and place settings to a bare minimum. Turn off the television or radio and keep the room quiet. She needs to be able to focus on what she is doing and that is eating and eating only.

This may seem silly to you. But remember, your brain is fully functional. That means your brain can assign value

Chapter 5 - Perceptions of Their World

to all the stimuli around you and decide what you need and don't need to be aware of. Stop now and listen to what you can hear. Do you hear the air conditioning blowing, traffic and cars outside, television's characters arguing or shouting to shooting at each other, neighbors going about their business, fire or police sirens, birds, the noise of a refrigerator?

Your brain can decide which noises you need to pay attention to now and which noises are not important and can be ignored. A person with Alzheimer's has a harder and harder time understanding and identifying the noise around us, so it is up to us to provide a calm and quiet environment, especially during meals and activities.

Given the deterioration of the brain, too much noise and stimulation is difficult for your loved one to decipher and be comfortable with. Eating should be q quiet time allowing the resident to focus solely on food. In facilities, look for a staff that is aware of the residents' need for quiet.

I was once asked to consult at a nursing home that had a special unit for mentally ill elderly persons who had now developed dementia as well. Walking into the unit during a meal, I was astonished to find the news being blared out over a television mounted on the wall. Several staff

Chapter 5 - Perceptions of Their World

members were standing and watching the news. Residents were yelling at each other, some fighting and some begging for food or attention. The noise level was impressive. After observing the residents and the noise levels, I walked over, reached up and turned the television off.

A resident seated in a wheelchair at the table under the television looked up at me and said "Thank you for doing that. I wanted to, but I couldn't reach it." Within five minutes, the entire atmosphere of the dining room had become calmer and quieter and residents were able to focus on eating.

The staff members standing and watching the television and not serving the residents however complained.

Nutrition and Hydration Changes

Additional visual problems can be identified if you realize Mom is only eating food on one side of the plate, or in a pie wedge shape. If this is happening, simply turn the plate to the next area and continue to do so until she has eaten all she wants.

This "pie wedge" eating is a sign, not that Mom loves potatoes and nothing else, but a sign that she can only

Chapter 5 - Perceptions of Their World

see a portion of the plate. Just turn the plate to allow her to see more of the food and continue to do so until she has finished her meal.

Alzheimer's people have a great difficulty tasting their food. As we age, there is a loss of taste buds in the tongue. But the loss is more dramatic for a person with Alzheimer's. The loss of taste is almost complete, with the exception of the taste for sweets. A resident can be presented with a beautiful meal and will not eat because she cannot taste the food.

I had a daughter tell me once that knowing her mother could taste and enjoy chocolate was a sure sign of a higher power because even with the loss of so many things, chocolate remained available as a comfort.

Think about the loss of taste this way: if you were presented with a beautiful meal and were extremely hungry, but the food tasted like cardboard, you probably wouldn't eat it. This is what faces your loved one. However, this dilemma can often be remedied by sprinkling sugar or applesauce on the food.

Giving snacks and foods an added sweet taste can often help slow the weight loss Alzheimer's people suffer. Remember you are striving for a total calorie count of more than 2800 calories per day and any way you can get

Chapter 5 - Perceptions of Their World

those calories in is helpful, especially as the disease progresses. Several pieces of candy throughout the day can help supplement the calorie count.

I have had families proudly tell me they were trying to force their mother to eat her food and since she was only interested in sweets, they made certain no sweets were available. The result was a mother who was dramatically losing weight.

If Mom wants to start with dessert or only eat dessert, do not allow this to become a battle. She needs calories, so go with the dessert. But try introducing a snack such as a sandwich later on or try her meal again if a half hour or so. But remember to sweeten the food and, just as you did with your children, praise her for eating, chewing and swallowing. Every bite counts.

Again, the use of alcohol and caffeine must stop with dementia. Your loved one's brain is under constant attack and can no longer process alcohol or caffeine. It is not morally or medically responsible or reasonable to give a beer or soda or glass of wine or cup of "real" coffee to a person with a damaged, two-pound brain.

Yet some assisted living companies will insist that without a doctor's order to stop giving alcohol, it is the person's right to drink whatever that person wants.

Chapter 5 - Perceptions of Their World

Remember, if a company states they offer a dementia specific program, then insist they offer a realistic dementia program with medically sound advice and experience. Dementia residents are not like other residents, it is up to the cognitive people to oversee the people with impaired cognition, and provide the safest and most homelike environment for them. If your loved one is living in your home, then you must be responsible to keep alcohol and caffeine out of harm's way.

Non-alcoholic and caffeine-free beverages are used as replacements. The person with dementia will not know the difference, especially as the disease progresses. Instead, it is the camaraderie of the social hour, or the special wine glass or the decorations on the fruit drink that give the impression she is having a "real" drink. That familiarity is the key.

The same is true with the morning newspaper or a book. Long after Mom can no longer read the newspaper, she may still look at it and turn the pages. This is because it is a familiar routine, a comfortable and familiar task. These are activities she enjoyed, old habits. But be aware, holding the newspaper and looking at the page is a far cry from reading and understanding the words and stories.

Chapter 5 - Perceptions of Their World

Chances are, she will continue to do familiar and life-long activities long after she truly understands the function or reason for those activities. And doing so will fool othose not familiar with your mom's disease process; into thinking Mom still has abilities she has lost.

Remember, in addition to calories, your mom also needs increased hydration to help her body avoid infection. If you or I were to stop drinking fluids for the rest of the day, we might get a headache, but tomorrow we would probably be fine.

Your mom however, could easily develop a urinary tract infection (UTI) by doing the same thing. You and I would know we had a UTI from a burning sensation when we urinate. Mom can't necessarily tell you she is burning. Instead you would watch for a sudden change in her behavior to alert you to the possibility of colds or infections.

Hearing Loss

There is some deterioration in hearing among the elderly. People with Alzheimer's also have difficulty with hearing, again, due to damage in the Temporal Lobe, as opposed to an actual hearing problem. The brain can no longer identify sound or the direction is originates from. As

Chapter 5 - Perceptions of Their World

the disease progresses, Alzheimer's residents often can't remember to wear hearing aids. Or Mom may find a hearing aid in her ear and toss it away. This is a very common thing to do and it doesn't help Mom to get angry with her or to blame her for throwing the hearing aid away. She is simply confused and doesn't remember what the item is or what it's function is.

Think about it like this, if you suddenly discovered a clump of something in your ear opening, you would probably throw it away as well. And given the price of hearing aids, this can become very expensive, so be aware that discarding items like eye glasses, dentures and hearing aids is another part of the disease process. Mom is not throwing things away to annoy you; she simply is unable to recognize the items for what they are.

As the brain deteriorates, the Temporal Lobe is attacked. It is one of the lobes that fill with cerebrospinal fluid and it controls language, the ability to smell and hearing. This loss of hearing can be dramatic and the challenges that result are equally dramatic.

Music and pitch of voice are better understood in lower tones. Higher pitches are lost to the ear. People who already have a hearing loss should be addressed directly and with a calm voice and calm face. Speak slowly and

Chapter 5 - Perceptions of Their World

clearly. Shouting at a person can be misinterpreted as anger and can cause Mom to have an outburst. But not enunciating words clearly enough can also cause an outburst.

I was speaking with a very interesting lady one day who has a hearing loss. I made certain I was amplifying my voice and keeping my face neutral as I shouted the conversation. I was concentrating to be sure my pitch was low and I was speaking clearly.

Mary had been a captain in the Women's Army Corps during World War II. She had been married to a colonel in the Army and they had three daughters. Mary's father had also served as a diplomat when Mary was a child.

"So Mary, your father was a diplomat in Belgium?" I asked. "Yes," she replied. "Papa was a smart man."

"And Mary," I continued loudly, "you learned to ice skate with your brothers there?"

"Yes, my brothers were wonderful skaters," she said.

"Now Mary," I said still speaking loudly and pleased with our conversation, "was your mother a good cook?"

"Crook!" Mary cried out. "My mother was not a crook. How dare you say that!"

Again I can only stress the importance of enunciating each word clearly.

Chapter 5 - Perceptions of Their World

Tactile Sensation

The sense of touch remains strong throughout life. Many Alzheimer's people lose most of their other senses, but retain touch. Items of different textures can be either stimulating or calming for them. Stroking a pet or animal fur can be soothing.

If you are afraid of your mom being scratched or grabbing the pet try using a rabbit fur item. A simple way to make one is to buy an old rabbit coat at the thrift store. Cut off one sleeve and stuff it with cloth and sew the ends shut. Mom may become calm or distracted while stroking the fur.

You may have also noticed your mom folding napkins or washcloths over and over or doing other repetitive movements like wiping the table or cleaning the counter. These are normal behaviors and can be used as activities to help calm your parent. Simply give her a basket of napkins to fold.

Other similar behaviors may include taking all the tissues out of the box and folding them again. She may then stuff the folded tissues into her clothing or place them in purses or drawers. Again, this folding and repetitive behavior is part of the disease process and should be allowed.

Chapter 5 - Perceptions of Their World

Giving Mom a basket of socks to sort is also a pastime that is safe and addresses the need to repeat motion and movement. Use socks of different textures and colors and allow for mistakes and always remember to praise effort and success.

Speech Changes

You have noticed Mom's aphasia, that is, the difficulty she has expressing herself with the right words and understanding the instructions she is given. You must begin to break tasks down into simple steps, so she can experience as much success as possible with activities of daily living. (ADLs are the everyday activities we do such as brushing our teeth, grooming, dressing, etc.) You should also give her praise throughout the task for her efforts and successes.

Caregivers should also be aware that Mom may misuse words in the same category to express herself, that is, she will pull words from a similar pool of words. For example, water or rain or river can translate into needing a drink or needing a bathroom. She may refer to her daughter as her sister or mother. She may refer to her son as her husband or brother.

Chapter 5 - Perceptions of Their World

In the early levels of the disease, she is confusing family terms with other words still used to describe family relationships. But as the disease progresses, she may begin to really believe a son is her father, simply based on a son who greatly favors her father's looks physically.

Persons who are bilingual will gradually lose their second language and remember only their first language. The memory is almost being removed in a reverse order, so what has been learned longest is retained longest. If a person learned Spanish or French as a second language, but learned English as their first language or native tongue, as the disease progresses, they will forget the Spanish or French and remember only the English.

This can be very challenging to children who never learned Mom's first language or to professional care givers in metropolitan areas.

For example, at one time I was the dementia director at a 60-bed unit in a large nursing home. Among the residents were a Russian, two Koreans, one Thai native, one Afghan, an Ethiopian, and an Albanian. The staff was challenged to use signs and communication books in the individual's native language to communicate with each person.

Chapter 5 - Perceptions of Their World

Of course as the disease progressed, the residents lost the ability to understand communication books and the staff fell back to relying on being certain the person had adequate nutrition and hydration, was not in discomfort or pain and did not develop any skin breakdowns.

But this doesn't mean new information cannot be learned. Procedural memory remains functional until the late stages of the disease. Procedural disease means Mom may learn where the dining room is when she is moved into a facility. But it doesn't mean she will always remember the location.

Pain and Temperature Changes

Alzheimer's persons are colder than normal elderly, but they may not know or recognize they are colder. In an aging person, the body core (the trunk area) is cooler, due to decreased circulation and physical changes and deterioration. Think about the body's natural cooling during aging. An 80-year-old person simply doesn't move as much as a four-year-old. This doesn't mean the older person's body temperature is 92 degrees instead of 98.6 degrees; rather, the cooling is happening by tiny changes in a degree.

Chapter 5 - Perceptions of Their World

But for the Alzheimer's patient, the core is at an even lower temperature. When I talk about a lower temperature, again, I mean only minuet changes, not entire degrees. The change is subtle, but it is there. The damaged brain cannot tell circulation to kick into gear, so the care giver must act instead. So since many Alzheimer's patients don't know they are colder or can't verbalize the need for a sweater, the care giver must remember and dress Mom accordingly.

I had one client Pat, who in August, with outside temperatures near 100 degrees, would be dressed in a turtleneck, sweater, pants and gloves. The rule of thumb is this, if I need a shirt, she may need a shirt and tee-shirt. If I need a shirt and tee-shirt, she may need a shirt, tee-shirt and sweater. Pat was an extreme example, but there is always one in every facility. Feel your mom's hands and feet. If her hands and feet are cold, she is cold and needs more clothing.

You may worry you will be unable to tell if your mom is in pain due to aphasia. Communication between humans is done in a number of ways and most of it does not involve speech. Remember when you brought home your newborn baby. That child could not speak, but you were still able to communicate. You could tell if your child was

Chapter 5 - Perceptions of Their World

sick or hungry or fussy, if your child was wet or soiled and needed to be changed. As the disease progresses, you will use those same skills to care for and communicate with your parent.

For example, you will always ask Mom if she is in pain when you suspect she is. As the disease progresses, you may not trust her answer (amnesia and aphasia). She may answer differently each time she is asked. Instead you will use the dementia pain scale to determine if Mom is hurting.

The dementia pain scale is similar to what you instinctively used with your child. You are watching for facial indicators (furrowed brows, frowning, wincing, a look of sadness), activity and movement changes (changes in breathing, tenseness, pacing, physical agitation or aggression), vocal (moaning, crying, pitch changes in her voice, cursing or verbal aggression), sleeping changes (curling up in a fetal position or kicking out, moving about or laying still), changes in personality and mood (sudden shifts in behavior or aggression or combativeness).

You know your mom better than anyone, so trust your instincts. A sudden change in behavior indicates Mom is feeling differently.

Chapter 5 - Perceptions of Their World

A sudden and dramatic change in cognition and behavior frequently indicates infection, usually a urinary tract infection (UTI). You are responsible for recognizing and assisting your loved one, so be aware of the behaviors indicating problems.

Communicating with Alzheimer's Patients

As you have learned, communication with a person with Alzheimer's becomes more and more challenging as the damage to the brain continues in the Frontal and Temporal Lobes. Depending upon the stage of the disease Mom is in, simple, clear instructions will be helpful. Repetition is a must. Professional care givers often report being tired of talking by the end of their shifts, because of the repetition of conversation and instructions to the residents.

First, prepare yourself to communicate. You should not be chewing gum or have candy in your mouth. Make sure you do not cover your mouth while you are talking. Just relax and know your time limits for every conversation. Remember, processing information, speech and language for a person with dementia is a challenge, so prepare to go slow.

Chapter 6 - Communicating with Alzheimer's Patients

Don't plan to stay for hours when visiting. Advanced dementia residents tire quickly and it is difficult for them to try and keep up. You should plan on limiting your visits from 15 minutes to an hour.

Prepare friends and other family members before they visit. Do not allow people to walk up and ask Mom "Do you remember me?" This is a generation of people with excellent social skills. Their social skills are so advanced; they can fool others into missing their cognition challenges because their skills at everyday conversations are so embedded.

But just think, have you ever been in a social or business setting where a person you know you should recognize asked you that same question? "Do you remember me?" It is embarrassing. For a person with dementia, it is up to us to supply many parts of the conversation to allow her to have maximum input and enjoyment.

Instead train your family and friends to approach conversations in this way: "Hi Mary. I'm Judy. I was your neighbor when you and your husband George lived at the beach. Your children were little and they played with my kids in the ocean." Or "Hi Grandma. I'm Becky, your granddaughter. Your son John is my father."

Chapter 6 - Communicating with Alzheimer's Patients

These clues in conversation allow for your mom's social skills to take over. She now knows who she is talking to and has a few clues to start with. This technique is much better than embarrassing her into guessing who a person is.

When you are sitting with your loved one and talking, feel free to hold her hand or touch her arm. Elderly people get touched less than any other group of people. We know human skin responds to touch, yet our older folks get fewer hugs than any other group. Bring lotion when you visit and offer Mom a hand or arm or leg or foot massage. The touch is therapeutic for both of you and the lotion helps her skin's integrity.

As time progresses, you will find yourself automatically slowing down when you are speaking with a person with dementia and these techniques will be rote.

Another challenge when doing this is to always remember you are communicating with an adult. You should avoid using "baby talk" or patronizing communication, but remember your tone.

As time passes, your tone will be similar to how you spoke to your children, soft and loving with gentle touches. Guard yourself and train other family members

Chapter 6 - Communicating with Alzheimer's Patients

or visiting friends to avoid speaking with an exaggerated slow rate, a higher pitch or an exaggerated intonation.

Remember to call the person by name frequently, but again do not use pet names unless you know the person well enough to know her nickname. Remember elderly women with dementia may not remember their husbands, depending upon the stage of dementia they are in.

So they may not respond to their married names, i.e. Mrs. Smith may not remember Mr. Smith. When she reaches that stage, calling Mrs. Smith by her first name is acceptable and less confusing to her.

But the person with Alzheimer's is never called "Grandma" by a care giver, unless she is the caregiver's grandmother. Pet names such as "sweetie" or "honey," "grandpa" or "Momma" should never be used in facilities.

Regardless of the stage Mom is currently in, it is always better to explain using short sentences. This gives Mom's brain a chance to process the information. But remember; never talk to her as though she were a child. She remains an adult. Use a clear and calm voice; describe what you are doing for and with Mom at each step.

For example dressing an adult with Level Five dementia would be something like: "Good Morning

Chapter 6 - Communicating with Alzheimer's Patients

Eunice. It's a beautiful day outside, but it's a little cold this morning. Let's get your blue sweater to put on. I'll help you. Put your right arm out first. Good. Now let's put the right sleeve on. Good, you are doing great. Let's bring the sweater around. Good. Now let's put your left hand through the sleeve. Good. You are doing so well. Soon we'll have this sweater on. Okay, that was wonderful. You always look so good in your blue sweater."

I realize this may sound corny, but you are basically breaking down each task into its' smaller components and giving praise and encouragement at each step. Everyone deserves praise for their efforts and when a person is fighting dementia, she deserves all the praise you can give. Giving praise also helps keep your temper from flaring when you become frustrated and angry with your mom's disease.

If you observe professional care givers (certified nursing assistants and nurses) the best ones always use this method for communicating - short sentences and lots of praise.

Be sure you are monitoring your nonverbal communication. Signs of impatience, annoyance, quick movements, etc., are noticeable, even to people with dementia, and those signs can be misinterpreted.

Chapter 6 - Communicating with Alzheimer's Patients

Encourage use of assistive or augmentative devices such as glasses, hearing aids, and communication boards with family and friends. Be prepared to repeat or write messages.

If you are a professional care giver, you should know the person's background. This will be a stimulus for conversation and help build rapport.

Make certain the physical environment is good before starting the conversation. Remember to look for adequate lighting, acoustics and seating. If you are visiting at a facility, you will probably want to go to a quiet area. Remember other people with dementia may be drawn to your group and want to be a part of the conversation. This can be very distracting for you and your loved one.

Alert the person that you are there and would like to talk. A touch on the shoulder or the hand, a handshake or a hug helps initiate this process. Break your conversations into smaller units for greater clarity and understanding. Remember to use short sentences, not long rambling sentences. Don't jump from topic to topic and give Mom background information. Orient her to the weather and month by conversation and memories.

For example if it is hot outside and your family always went to the beach in the summer, discuss those

Chapter 6 - Communicating with Alzheimer's Patients

memories. If a certain season meant certain foods she cooked or family events, discuss those with her. Keep similar topics together and try not to jump from one topic to another. Use a familiar vocabulary, words and phrases she would understand. It will also help her if you use nouns rather than pronouns.

Supplement the conversation with appropriate gestures, pantomime and pointing. Watch how we actually talk to each other. Most of our conversations are movements and gestures, facial expressions, etc.

Try to avoid asking open-ended questions, unless you are supplying the answers. As the disease progresses, it will be harder and harder for her to answer questions. Try something more like this: "Hi Dad, I'm your daughter Sally. Did you have breakfast today? It looks like you've had a good breakfast, eggs and pancakes and bacon. I know you love bacon."

This way you've asked a question, but keyed Dad on how to answer and join the conversation.

Remember to pause frequently and check for comprehension. Do not use abstract thoughts and concepts and encourage conversation about memories your loved one can provide. As times this may be frustrating, but as the disease progresses and she can no

Chapter 6 - Communicating with Alzheimer's Patients

longer have conversations, you'll remember these times fondly. Reflect on your loved one's expressed feelings. Keep communication as enjoyable as possible and encourage reminiscence.

Sit at an arm's length and face the person at eye level. If she is in a wheelchair, you will need to bend over to face her or sit to allow her to see your face while you all are speaking. If hearing is an issue, remember to face the person and lean forward to increase volume, but do not give the appearance of shouting, as this can be misinterpreted as anger. Remember to use her communication board. Black ink is easiest to see, so keep a spare pen available.

Eliminate background noise, for example turn off the television, radio, etc. and move to a quiet place if in a group setting. Remember to maintain the social roles of conversation. Encourage your mom to talk and listen to what she says, even when it no longer makes sense. At that point, you respond to the tone. If she is talking and doesn't make any sense, but she is laughing, then you should be laughing with her.

In my first job as a social worker in a nursing home, I knew a man who had a massive stroke. Charlie had been a farmer and a rancher all his life. Now, he could only say

Chapter 6 - Communicating with Alzheimer's Patients

two words and those two words were not socially acceptable and he would not say them at social events. He would just sit quietly. But if you ignored the two words and listened to his tone and inflection, you could still have a meaningful conversation with him. I will use two other words to replace the words Charlie had to use.

The conversation would go like this: "Say Charlie, did you see the price of cattle in the paper this week? I tell you I don't know how the poor old ranchers are going to make a living this year."

"Apple orange, apple orange," Charlie would reply, shaking his head up and down for "Yes." Here his voice tone and intonation would really get going. "Apple orange, APPLE ORANGE, apple orange, apple orange."

"Yeah, I know what you mean. The ranchers are going to be hurting come winter time and time to buy feed."

Charlie would shake his head again in agreement and use his hands to emphasize, "Oh apple orange, apple orange, apple orange."

So we had a conversation and we both understood what we were talking about, but I think we probably alarmed others around us.

Shaking hands is another one of the ways we communicate with others, especially this generation of

Chapter 6 - Communicating with Alzheimer's Patients

elderly. A simple handshake can communicate a great deal of information to the resident and allow for a quick and positive interaction. Shaking hands can also allow you to redirect your loved one away from others or distract her if she is becoming combative.

Asking your mom "Why?" she did or didn't do something can be a frustrating and negative experience as it requires a higher level of brain function. Your mom can be embarrassed because she doesn't know the answer. Rewording the question and understanding that her behavior is a result of the damage being caused by the disease can mean a more positive experience for her and a less frustrating one for you.

Social skills will remain strong with your mom until the very end of the disease. For most people, social skills begin very early in life. After parents teach a child to say "Mommy" and "Daddy", they begin to teach saying "Please" and "Thank you" and "You're welcome." These skills can remain after other skills are lost and can be used to provide a positive experience for you and your loved one. Remember, as long as I am polite, she is polite.

People with dementia don't respond well to arguments because they can't use higher functioning to make their

Chapter 6 - Communicating with Alzheimer's Patients

point. Arguing is more likely to frustrate the care giver and cause the Alzheimer's patient to react negatively. Alzheimer's persons may not be able to determine why someone is shouting, but the very action and noise may cause a negative event for both parties. Persons suffering from a hearing loss may also interpret shouting as anger and respond accordingly.

People with Alzheimer's frequently become paranoid because they don't understand their environment. Most people would exhibit some form of paranoia if their surrounding environment did not make sense to them. Not being able to understand the language, not being able to hear the words being spoken, not understanding why a bath is needed, eating food that is not what one remembers or can taste, being in a place that doesn't feel familiar, all these things can lead to paranoia.

7

Global Deterioration Scale Characteristics

While we most often hear about Alzheimer's, currently another 2 to 4 million or so families in this country are often confronted with additional or other types of dementias.

Even though there are a variety of dementias, all the dementias can be classified by stage on a seven level measurement of behaviors called the Global Deterioration Scale. This scale determines individual stages based on behaviors, characteristic signs, specific losses of abilities and symptoms exhibited by the affected person.

The major difference between Alzheimer's and another types of dementia, like Vascular Dementia for example, is that the Alzheimer's person will follow the stages, one through seven, as though she were on a slippery slope, while the vascular dementia person may have a stroke or

Chapter 7 – The Global Deterioration Scale Characteristics

someother type of event severe enough to cause her to skip one of more stages.

This type of dementia may be referred to as a "side-step" dementia because the person has a significant decline in her abilities and then her cognition and her health stabilize, and then there is another event and another major decline in abilities. This person is "side-stepping" through the stages rather than continually declining on a daily basis.

The seven stages or levels are divided into early, middle and late dementia. Early includes Level One and Level Two, middle is Level Three and Four and late covers Levels Five, Six and Seven. The late stage is also referred to as the "terminal stage" as this is where death normally occurs.

It is important to remember that not all persons will progress through their specific dementia at the same rate of time, and not all will display all of the characteristics present for each specific stage.

There is enough current research to support estimated times for the length of each stage, but these times vary based on the individual's own health.

For example a person in otherwise good health will progress differently than a person with multiple health

Chapter 7 – The Global Deterioration Scale Characteristics

complications such as hypertension, end stage renal failure, cancer, etc.

It can be difficult to predict the length of time a patient with Alzheimer's disease will stay in a specific level or stage. One person may stay in one stage for a longer period of time than the scale estimates and then that person may quickly progress through the other stages. For example, a person may take years to reach Level Five and then quickly progress over several months to the end of the disease. The length of time for each stage can vary greatly from person to person.

However, symptoms seem to progress in a recognizable pattern and the seven stages provide a framework for understanding and tracking the disease progression in a person. It is important to remember the stages are not uniform in every patient and the stages often overlap.

Early Stage – Level One and Level Two

The early stage of dementia is believed to last from two to four years. Unfortunately, a diagnosis of dementia is usually not made at this time because there are 100 other disorders which present with the same signs and symptoms in the first stage.

Chapter 7 – The Global Deterioration Scale Characteristics

This early stage is marked by gradual and very subtle changes that occur slowly over time. A person's spouse, family or friends usually do not recognize anything is wrong or attributes cognitive changes to stress, lack of sleep, job, getting older, etc. And the person is usually very good at concealing and compensating for deficiencies during the first stage.

The person may do very well in social situations and in a normal nonspecific conversation. Remember that a great many of our conversations are nonspecific. The conversations begin with a standard greeting that everyone is familiar with such as, "Hello. How are you?"

We have been trained since we learned to speak to respond to that phrase and question and dozens more like it. It is important to remember in every culture, social skills are taught from a very young age. This teaching of social skills is a universal concept. And since Alzheimer's is typically destroying the brain's memories in a reverse order, this long term memory of social skill knowledge is retained and used until the final stage of the disease when speech is lost.

It is only when you ask a very specific question, such as her age, the year, the date, or events from the past week or day , i.e. what was eaten for dinner, who called

Chapter 7 – The Global Deterioration Scale Characteristics

on the telephone, etc., that there are indications her cognition is impaired.

Even at this early stage, most people will try to hide the disease. Your loved one may use humor to answer questions which are confusing, which can lead to a misconception by friends and family the patient is actually quite "with it" and the humorous answer proves it. If however, you continue to question the person to give you a correct answer; the result can be a frustrated and angry outburst.

Most people are very aware in the second level of Alzheimer's that they are having difficulty with their memory. They may display symptoms of depression over their memory loss in this second level or depressive symptoms may not present until a later stage of the disease. Depression is considered a likely part of the disease because the person is aware she is no longer remembering things she should know, like her name, her children's names, her spouse, her address, what she did this morning or yesterday, etc.

Level One

Level One is the normal stage of cognition for humans. It means you know who you are and where you are. You

Chapter 7 – The Global Deterioration Scale Characteristics

are alert and oriented to person, time and place. Your thought processes are logical and your cognition is intact and operating normally. Remember, dementia is not a normal part of the aging process, it is a disease. Most of us will live and die, still knowing who we are experiencing only the normal forgetfulness that all human beings exhibit.

It is important when you are a family member dealing with a person with Alzheimer's that you understand how the brain responds to stimuli and short term and long term memory. The normal forgetfulness and processing of the brain can "trick" you into thinking that you also have dementia. Remember, the brain assigns value to all the information around it. If it did not, you would be overwhelmed by all the stimuli around you.

One way to see how your brain works is to think about driving in congested traffic. In heavily populated areas, people are frequently driving on streets and interstate highways with thousands of other drivers. Your brain automatically assigns value to the cars around you.

It decides which car to pay attention to, which car to then ignore because it no longer needs to track that vehicle. The brain determines which car needs to be watched because it is turning or slowing or speeding by

Chapter 7 – The Global Deterioration Scale Characteristics

you. Your brain is aware and watching for traffic lights, policemen, wrecks, cars being driven erratically, etc. And as soon as the brain determines it no longer needs information on a specific car, it dismisses that information.

The same thing happens to your brain all day long. If you get up from your chair and go to another room to get something, but then can't remember why you went into the other room, your brain is not demented; it simply didn't assign value to the information. In other words, your brain didn't think what you were looking for was important enough to remember.

When you look up a telephone number and forget that number before you can even dial it, again, that is not dementia. The brain simply decided the telephone number was a number you would never again need or use, so it immediately discarded the information.

And when you can't remember someone's name, but you can "see" the face and "feel" the name on your tongue, it doesn't mean you have dementia. It just means you filed the information in a different manner than you are now attempting to access it. Think of the brain's memory like a computer. If I filed Brad's name in the Jennifer file and now I'm looking for him in Angelina's file, the computer won't be able to locate Brad. The difference

Chapter 7 – The Global Deterioration Scale Characteristics

between the brain and the computer however, is that the brain will continue to try and solve the problem. That's why about 20 minutes later you will suddenly remember Brad

Level Two – Two to Four Years

Level Two is Very Mild Cognitive Decline – Forgetfulness. This is the beginning of dementia, where the disease starts to affect the brain's operations. The changes in each stage now are divided into cognitive, affective and physical. Cognitive changes are changes in perception and awareness. Affective changes are changes in emotions and feelings. Physical changes are the observable changes we can see in a person's physical condition.

Cognitive changes include memory loss – especially of recent events and new information, an uncertainty and hesitancy in initiating behaviors and actions, a visibly lessened ability to perform simple tasks, an increased loss of reason, logic and judgment and difficulty focusing attention or a decreased attention span. Amnesia and aphasia are present and observable.

The affective changes include a decreased interest in environment and present affairs, a type of social

Chapter 7 – The Global Deterioration Scale Characteristics

withdrawal. The person may exhibit an indifference to the normal courtesies of social life. There is a loss of initiative and sense of humor. Some people may have a noticeable personality change. The person exhibits a lack of spontaneity, often seen as absent-mindedness, a decreased ability to concentrate, and a slower and decreased initiative drive or lack of initiative. This person may also exhibit an overall dull affect or lack of emotion on her face.

A fastidious person may become slightly more careless in her appearance and actions. Her family may witness an emotional instability. The two most common emotions are depression, because the person is aware she is forgetful, or anger and/or frustration because she cannot remember or do the things the way she was accustomed to doing them.

There may begin to be marital problems along with personality changes, primarily due to amnesia events. There are very few physical changes at this stage. The person appears fine and may have such good health that she can go out and run a mile, come home and forget where she put her tennis shoes. She may have slight weakness or slower movements and she may have a small amount of muscle twitching.

Chapter 7 – The Global Deterioration Scale Characteristics

By the end of Level Two, the person is beginning to perform poorly at work. She might forget to perform tasks that were routine in her daily life. She may be unable to add or subtract a figure correctly, have difficulty organizing times and dates, and may be in jeopardy of retaining her job. Upon questioning by friends or a physician, she will have an appropriate interest and concern about the symptoms beginning to present themselves.

Middle Stage – Levels Three and Four - Two to Twelve Years

The diagnosis of some type of dementia is usually made here. Families may be relieved to know that the relative has a "disease" and is not crazy, but difficulties in the family can also arise here when one child or another family member refuses to recognize or accept the disease.

Signs, symptoms and behaviors are beginning to be magnified many times in Level Three. The person is usually taken to a doctor, because the family is aware of her memory loss and is beginning to recognize her decline in intellectual functioning is too pronounced to be "normal."

Chapter 7 – The Global Deterioration Scale Characteristics

During the Middle Stage the person can fluctuate from one stage to another throughout the day. Most of the time, the person is unaware she is making errors. She is also unaware she may be "filling in" with sounds instead of words during conversations. She is unaware she may be of losing her train of thought during conversation and it becomes more difficult for her to even hold a conversation.

It is important to remember that during a conversation, she may present well, but realistically may not be certain as to who you are.

She may begin wandering, sometimes for hours, until she becomes tired and recognizes she is tired. It will be difficult for her to sit still.

She will exhibit a loss of reasoning powers. She will be aware only of the present and will be unaware of what happened yesterday.

She will have difficulty planning for tomorrow. She will be largely unaware of her surroundings and her generalized confusion will lead to increased anxiety.

She will begin to ask the same question repeatedly or repeat stories constantly (amnesia).

Chapter 7 – The Global Deterioration Scale Characteristics

She will begin to exhibit an inability to retain or process information, as the loss of short term memory is now present and evident to others.

During the Middle Stage a few brain pathways and personality traits remain intact and undamaged.

She may begin to accept the fact that she is sick, but she will begin to take greater measures to hide her deficits. She will accept reassurance from her caregiver, but will also become depressed and withdrawn.

Level Three

Level Three is Mild Cognitive Decline – Early Confusional Stage. Characteristics being monitored from the Global Deterioration Scale include one or more of the following: she may have gotten lost traveling to a familiar place, co-workers are aware of an increasingly poor job performance, word and name finding difficulties are evident to intimates, she will retain little information when reading a book or passage, she may show increased difficulty remembering names of new acquaintances, she may lose a valuable object, she will exhibit mild to moderate anxiety and she will exhibit a decreased performance level in social and employment settings.

Chapter 7 – The Global Deterioration Scale Characteristics

And she will now begin to deny deficits and begin to attempt to cover up memory glitches.

Her recent memory loss will begin to affect job performance. She will wonder what she was just told to do. Her confusion about places means she may get lost on the way to work or when coming home from work.

She will lose the initiative to start new things and she will lose her spontaneity, that "spark of life," as her mood and personality begins to change. She will become anxious about her symptoms and will begin to avoid people.

Routine chores will take longer. She will have trouble paying bills and handling money. She may pay the same bills several times over, or not pay the bills for three months.

Her poor judgment will lead to poor decisions. She will have difficulty remembering telephone numbers. She will arrive at the wrong time or the wrong place and will constantly check the calendar or make lists. Family members report that "Mother's not the same – she's withdrawn, disinterested." She may spend all day making dinner, but forget to serve several courses.

The following is a generalized list of the decline in abilities, as well as some of the behavioral symptoms: she

Chapter 7 – The Global Deterioration Scale Characteristics

will have difficulty in understanding a story or a joke and difficulty in telling a story correctly, she will lose her train of thought in the middle of the sentence, misuse a word, substitute one word for another, lose track of money or check book balances, misplace belongings or lose them, her forgetfulness will be viewed as being more than normal, her conversations will be less appropriate, including the wrong response to what is said to her or saying what she is thinking, confusion during meals, confusion in unfamiliar or familiar situations.

She may change her manner of dress, including unmatched clothing, no jacket when it's cold, layering clothing, an inability to find something when it is in its proper place, taking longer than normal to complete a task or show an inability to complete a task.

She may exhibit changes in her sleep pattern, show poor judgment in decision making or be unable to make a decision. She may have small mishaps with the car such as denting a fender on her way into the garage, forgetting where car is parked or have accidents with the car. She may be unable to follow simple directions when driving or walking.

She may exhibit inappropriate mood changes and may present with a flaccid facial appearance. She may answer

Chapter 7 – The Global Deterioration Scale Characteristics

"yes" or "no" to questions, instead of discussing something in a conversation. She may use humor to deflect a question she can't answer, which can further confuse families or convince them she is really "okay" cognitively. She may become agitated for no apparent reason or become belligerent.

She may begin avoiding people outside the home, withdraw from activities, or forget an invitation to an event and accuse the family of not including her in family events.

She will begin sleeping more than usual, have a change in her normal appetite, exhibit wide mood swings, poor coordination or balance (apraxia) and have an increase or decrease in her sexual desires and behaviors. She will become disoriented to time or place.

Level Four

Level Four is Moderate Cognitive Decline – Late Confusional. Cognitive changes include obvious defects in memory, retention, and recall. Her recent memory is the first to go. She will have difficulty concentrating; she will easily lose her train of thought and will exhibit hesitation with her verbal responses.

Chapter 7 – The Global Deterioration Scale Characteristics

She will forget appointments and socially significant events. She will also forget to initiate or complete normal routines, including health and hygiene measures.

At night she will exhibit aimless wandering or restlessness. She will confuse day and night as her nocturnal clock is damaged. She will lose items and claim they are stolen. She will have hallucinations and may exhibit inappropriate social behaviors. She will have an increased dependence on significant others, have role reversal or she will become socially isolated.

She will be unable to recognize herself in the mirror. She may even stand in front of a mirror in the bathroom or bedroom and talk to herself and not realize she is actually talking to herself. And if she doesn't recognize *herself,* you can see how she would not recognize her family, neighbors and friends, etc.

She will have a greater challenge understanding or expressing language (aphasia). She will be unable to attach meaning to sensory impression. She will be unable to do math calculations (amnesia). She will have difficulty reading or writing. She may however hold a newspaper and appear to be reading.

Apraxia (poor muscle coordination) will become apparent to observers. Apraxia can affect even healthy

Chapter 7 – The Global Deterioration Scale Characteristics

older adults who don't maintain an exercise regime, but not the same as a person with dementia. A normally aging adult needs to continue to be mobile to maintain balance and function, while a person with dementia loses balance and function due to damage and the loss of brain structures.

Her symptoms will include an increasing loss of memory, greater confusion and a shorter attention span. She will have problems recognizing close friends and her family.

Repetitive statements and movements will be noticeable by others. She may have occasional muscle twitches or jerking and perceptual motor problems. She will have difficulty organizing thoughts or thinking logically and won't be able to find the right words, so she will makes up stories to fill in blanks.

She will have problems with reading, writing, numbers and calculations. She may become suspicious, irritable, fidgety, teary or silly. She will begin to fear bathing. She will begin to need fulltime supervision. She may undress at inappropriate times or at the wrong place.

She won't remember family or friends visiting immediately after they leave. She may accuse families of failing to include her in events because she doesn't

Chapter 7 – The Global Deterioration Scale Characteristics

remember being invited or attending. She will sleep more often, especially during the day.

She may exhibit a huge appetite for junk food and other peoples' food; but then forget when her last meal was eaten, and then she will gradually lose all interest in food.

Late Stage – Levels Five, Six and Seven – One to Nine Years

This begins the Late Stage. Cognitive changes include little or no response to stimuli, an inability to perform purposeful movements or recognize others – even family members.

Affective changes include lethargy and a flat affect or the lack of visible emotion on the face. There will be little to no movement of the eyebrows, mouth, cheeks, etc. The face is "flat" in appearance and without emotion.

Physical changes include weight loss, even with an increased appetite. She may experience seizures, incontinence, extreme psychomotor retardation (the inability to move with coordination or purpose), and a greater susceptibility to injury and infection. In the final stage, she may groan, cry out or grunt. She will require total care to dress, bath and groom herself. Aphasia, agnosia, apraxia and amnesia are complete.

Chapter 7 – The Global Deterioration Scale Characteristics

Late Stage – Level Five – One to Three Years

Level Five is Moderately Severe Cognitive Decline – Early Dementia. This is typically when a family requires the need of a nursing or assisted living facility. Their loved one now requires total physical or nursing care or 24-hour monitoring for safety.

Interactions with a person in this stage will reveal: During an interview, the person may be unable to recall a major relevant aspect of current life, e.g. an address or telephone number of many years, the names of close family members (such as grandchildren), or the name of the high school or college from which he/she graduated (amnesia). However, she should know her name, her spouses' name and her children's' names.

Persons at this stage will retain knowledge of many major facts regarding themselves or others. In social conversation, this person continues to present as a fully functioning person.

Frequently there is some disorientation to time (year, date, day, week, season) or to place. An educated person may have difficulty counting backwards from 40 by 4s or from 20 by 2s.

Chapter 7 – The Global Deterioration Scale Characteristics

Social skills are good and demonstrated in use; however the person may use humor to sidestep a question requiring more detailed knowledge or higher cognitive ability. The person may become argumentative, upset or combative if pressed to answer questions beyond her capabilities at this point. She will revert to humor to disguise deficits.

Immediate memory (about five minutes) is relatively impaired. Speech and language skills are still functional, although information, questions and stories will be repeated. She typically will enjoy reminiscing conversations about "the good old days."

She will still have a sense of awareness, but she is "lost in time." She will have knowledge of past, present and future events. Her perception of reality is based on misperceptions. This person retains the ability to form a thought, plan an action and follow-through, so wandering is a very real danger or concern.

This person will continue to believe she still has responsibilities. The responsibilities may be work-related or family/housekeeping-related. For example, she may want to leave to go to work or check on her family or her children.

Chapter 7 – The Global Deterioration Scale Characteristics

Normal behaviors at this stage are: This person can no longer survive without some assistance, but will still look "normal." An outsider or family member with little contact would have difficulty believing there are serious cognitive difficulties. It is not unusual for this person to hold a newspaper or book as though still able to read and comprehend the meaning of the articles. This person should still be able to read some words, but not necessarily make meaning of the sentences.

This person will wear clothing and supportive appliances such as dentures, hearing aids, eye glasses, jewelry, scarves and a hat. Women will carry a purse and men will carry a wallet. Typically, men will not leave the residence without some amount of cash (even a single dollar), whereas women will leave with no money and just their purse.

This person will be resistant to care giving, as she does not believe she needs assistance from others. Activities of daily living are relatively intact, but supervision is needed for eating, toileting, bathing, grooming and dressing.

This person may resist bathing and insist she has already bathed. First signs of combativeness may occur here when care givers insist on giving her a bath.

Chapter 7 – The Global Deterioration Scale Characteristics

This person will exhibit a pattern of wandering with a purpose (actively wandering), i.e., exit-seeking or elopement or running away with a purpose, such as "I'm going to feed my babies" or "I'm going to see my sick mamma." She may start to go somewhere and lose her train of thought. This behavior may be perceived as purposeless wandering, which is a behavior associated with Level Six of the disease process.

Delusional behavior, suspicious behavior and anxiety related to short-term memory loss causing misperceptions, are present. She may accuse family members or care givers of theft, usually because her memory is impaired and she doesn't remember where an item has been placed.

The person may also accuse the care giver of attempting to harm her, because of confusion about the activity being performed, i.e. bathing can be interpreted as an assault or attack (agnosia, amnesia and apraxia).

Tearfulness, depression and catastrophic outbursts can be present.

This person retains her own agenda and insight into situations. Her belief about her surroundings is very real to her, regardless of how nonsensical the care giver may perceive the situation.

Chapter 7 – The Global Deterioration Scale Characteristics

Environmental stimuli can prompt behavior. Too much background noise or too much movement, too many people or cars or city lights, can be upsetting to this person. Shouting can be misinterpreted as anger and cause her to become physically or verbally combative.

This person needs validation of his/her reality and feelings. If the person is seeking a dead relative for example, she is missing that person and no longer has the memory of that loved one's death. She should not be corrected about the loved one's death, but the care giver can talk about the missed loved one and in doing so, often sooth the distress the person is feeling. After a few minutes, the care giver can attempt to redirect the conversation.

Remember her reality is your reality. To become aggravated and insist on telling her that her husband or mother or child is dead is devastating and hurtful. She will have the same response as the first time she found out her loved one had died, she will once again experience that terrible pain of loss.

Sometimes adult children become upset when a demented mother doesn't remember their father and they insist on telling her that he has died. They may do this to ease their own grief or to get what they perceive is an

Chapter 7 – The Global Deterioration Scale Characteristics

appropriate grief response from her, but to tell your mother again and again that your father has died is wrong. The "mother" you are seeing **not** react to your father's death is not really your mother, it is the disease process and that is what you must remember. It is one of the parts of life the disease makes so difficult for the family.

This person believes she doesn't really live here; instead she is "just visiting." "Sun downing" syndrome will now become evident in the afternoon hours. Sundowning is a disease process in which the person begins to actively or inactively wander.

Actively wandering means Mom is wandering with a purpose. She believes she needs to leave the house to go pick up her children or to return home to her parent's house. Inactive wandering means she is moving around, but isn't able to say where she is going or why she needs to leave.

There are numerous theories about Sundowning's causation. Some believe it is caused by Restless Leg Syndrome. Others believe the change of shifts in a facility trigger the need to leave. I think it is related to a human history of movement and activity in the afternoon hours. As humans, since the earliest time, we have changed our

Chapter 7 – The Global Deterioration Scale Characteristics

activity in the afternoon. We stopped hunting and made a shelter for the night. Or we stopped farming and returned to our hut.

In the past century, our parents returned home in the afternoon from their jobs. As children and throughout our educational years, we left our schools and returned home. As adults we left our jobs and returned home. It is ingrained in humans from childhood to leave one place in the afternoon and go to another place to prepare an evening meal and sleep.

Sundowning is especially challenging for care givers. Mom may be quite insistent about leaving, because she truly believes she needs to leave. Her determination to go home or go pick up her children is based in her reality. She is just as serious about leaving as you would be if you knew you needed to get your children or check on a loved one.

Sometimes talking to her about how much she cares about the person or people she wants to go to will calm her when she wants to leave. You may be able to redirect her with another activity. And sometimes just taking her for a short walk will burn up that excess energy. But be aware that Sundowning is very difficult for some people and very frustrating for care givers. At this stage, Mom

Chapter 7 – The Global Deterioration Scale Characteristics

should still be able to toilet and eat independently, but may have difficulty choosing the proper clothing to wear. Remember that eating independently and safely preparing foods are two different activities. She is at risk for eating food that has spoiled or turning on the stove and forgetting it is on.

Incontinent episodes may occur on occasion, and should prompt a check for urinary tract infection (UTI) by the care givers. Sudden and aggressive changes in behavior should be monitored by the physician to rule out UTIs, colds or other infections which can cause delirium.

She may enjoy folding clothing such as napkins, Kleenex, towels, etc., and may perform this activity for hours or throughout the day.

Depression can become an issue as this person is still aware that she is losing her abilities. In this stage she will admit to being afraid because she can no longer remember her family. She may make statements to others that she believes she is a burden to others and that she wishes to die.

Finally, the Level Five person is easily annoyed with Level Six persons. The Level Five person tends to regard Level Six people as petulant children who should be disciplined. Contrastingly, Level Five persons view Level

Chapter 7 – The Global Deterioration Scale Characteristics

Seven persons as being aged and ill and respond more appropriately to them.

This person's brain weighs approximately two to two and one-half pounds.

Level 6 – One to Three Years

Level Six is Severe Cognitive Decline – Middle Dementia. Interactions with a person in this stage will reveal: During an interview, this person will be largely unaware of all recent events and experiences in her life (amnesia). She will forget the name of the spouse or adult child care giver upon whom she is entirely dependent upon for survival. She may continue to know her own name. She is in her own world and largely unaware of others.

This person's speech and language deficits are more pronounced (aphasia). She will not be able to think abstractly or comprehend deficits. She will revert to her mother tongue.

This person will retain some knowledge of her life, but the information on recall is sketchy at best. Her recall is better in past events of her life, although she will discuss those events as if they are occurring in present time. She will be generally unaware of her surroundings, i.e. what

Chapter 7 – The Global Deterioration Scale Characteristics

year it is, what season, month, day of the week, etc. She will have less than five minutes of short-term memory.

She will demonstrate the loss of peripheral vision. She can be startled by persons walking up behind or to the side of her, because she does not see them until they suddenly "appear" next to her.

She will begin to experience a loss of depth perception. This loss will continue until her visual perception of her environment is flat, like a photograph, rather than three dimensional. She will tap the floor with her foot when the texture or color of the floor changes (carpet to wood floor, crossing into an elevator, stepping from the sidewalk to pavement) because to her that change appears to be a hole.

The tapping is to make certain the flooring is solid and she won't fall. These changes in vision are related to the damage being done to the brain and not to damage to the eye or the lack of glasses.

She will have difficulty counting backwards from 10 and counting to 10 from one.

This person will require assistance with all ADLs and will frequently become aggressive or combative during those ADLs. To complete any ADLs on her own, she will need a visual "jump-start."

Chapter 7 – The Global Deterioration Scale Characteristics

This person's diurnal rhythm is now greatly disturbed and she may sleep during the day and stay awake through the night or may require 16 or more hours of sleep and then stay awake for 18 or more hours. Some persons will stay awake for two or more days at a time before requiring sleep, or this person may fall asleep during meals or while doing activities.

Normal behaviors at this stage are: she will now look "unfinished." She will not want to change her clothing and will frequently layer clothing. Her face will begin to have an even more flat look or affect.

Interaction with her will reveal serious cognitive decline and loss of abilities. She will no longer recognize or be able to use common objects (agnosia). For example, a person with Alzheimer's may use a spoon instead of a fork, a razor instead of a toothbrush, a trash can instead of a urinal, a scarf instead of a napkin.

She will usually retain social skills, but the use of those skills is rudimentary, i.e., she will be unable to converse after social pleasantries are exchanged. She will tend to talk using social clichés, without really understanding the meaning. She cannot initiate conversation or engage in conversation regarding recent events.

Chapter 7 – The Global Deterioration Scale Characteristics

This person now becomes a real risk for falls as the deterioration of the brain impairs the ability to coordinate muscular movement and coordination (apraxia). Her posture, gait and balance are all affected and become quite pronounced by the end of this stage.

She will nonetheless restlessly pace about, increasing the need for calories and rest periods. Or she may refuse to walk or lose interest in walking or no longer remember how to walk (apraxia).

She will continue to be able to distinguish familiar persons in the environment, but she is unable to recall names properly. She may call her son by the wrong name or may introduce him as her "father," or her "brother," or her "uncle," or her "sister," etc. She is pulling names from the same pool of words for family members. Likewise, she may talk about rain or water or thirsty or storm and mean she needs to be toileted.

She will remove accessories such as eye glasses, dentures, hearing aids, splints, braces, wound dressings, shortly after putting them on. She will most likely throw the objects away or place them in an odd area as she discards them (agnosia).

She becomes incontinent of bladder and possibly bowel during this stage. She is generally unaware of the

Chapter 7 – The Global Deterioration Scale Characteristics

need to urinate. She requires travel assistance, but occasionally, she will display the ability to travel to familiar locations.

She will now frequently exhibit personality and emotional changes. Common changes include delusional behavior (she may accuse her spouse of being an imposter and react violently towards him) or she may demonstrate obsessive symptoms, such as repeatedly performing cleaning activities.

She will have anxiety, agitation and previously nonexistent violent behavior may occur. Her cognitive impairment can be seen because she cannot carry a thought long enough to determine a purposeful course of action.

She will complete activities "my way." She does not believe she has "any responsibilities." She is unconcerned about her whereabouts and collects "things" during the day. To avoid combative outbursts, try trading for objects rather than taking objects from her.

This person may develop a fear of being alone. She will frequently search for social contact. If she is moved to a facility, she may confuse another resident with an old friend and spend most of the day with him or her.

Chapter 7 – The Global Deterioration Scale Characteristics

This isnot an unusual event to have happen and it makes adjusting to a new place much easier.

At this stage, a person will nurture Level Seven persons and listen to Level Five persons.

This person's brain weighs approximately one and one-half to two pounds.

Level 7 – 1 to 3 years – Terminal Stage

Level Seven is Very Severe Cognitive Decline – Late Dementia. At this stage, the person looks abnormal. She will be unable to initiate conversation or interactions with others.

Speech and language deficits (aphasia) are evident. In conversing with this person or when attempting to engage this person, only a brief attention span is evident. She will be unable to recognize familiar persons or use common objects (agnosia).

She will begin to have the onset of weight loss and will require more and more assistance with feeding, up to total assistance. As the disease progresses, she will forget how to chew food or swallow food and will need assistance and prompting to eat.

As the brain continues to deteriorate, she will begin pocketing food between her cheeks and gums and will

Chapter 7 – The Global Deterioration Scale Characteristics

need to be assessed for a change in diet texture (pureed food and thickened liquids) to avoid aspirating on food. She will forget she is hungry or thirsty and will be unable to swallow food safely. She may drool, as the swallow reflex has diminished (apraxia).

The person may seek and search for immediate sensory gratification, i.e. if it looks good, tastes good, and feels good, she will do it. This is a self-stimulatory activity. She may exhibit hyper-oral activity in the beginning, placing anything in her mouth.

She will suffer significant posture changes, including losing the ability to walk, hold her head up or maintain her balance when sitting (apraxia).

She may attempt to remove her clothing, regardless of the temperature and she will fidget when sitting or laying down.

She will lose her ability to see the environment around her, including a loss of 3-D Vision. Everything will appear flat, like a photograph.

She will become completely incontinent, although the 90-second rule may continue to work within one hour of meals, for a time. She may become even more resistive to care giving or will become totally placid, almost semi-comatose.

Chapter 7 – The Global Deterioration Scale Characteristics

She will be unable to say her name, her parents' name or recognize her family (amnesia, aphasia and apraxia). Her eyes will have a vacant look without focus and she will maintain a flat affect, finally losing her ability to smile. She will be unaware of danger.

She may rock or have hyper-oral activity. Hyper-oral activity means she may try to eat anything she can get into her mouth, including trash and feces.

She may utter a few non-meaningful words or non-words, or vocalize by sound in response to painful stimuli, or she may remain mute while in pain.

Care givers should rely upon the scale for dementia pain to determine if she is hurting, i.e., facial cues, wincing, sharp breath intakes, etc.

She will fail to comprehend spoken language, but may show awareness for simple gestures, pantomimes, facial expressions, familiar musical tunes, environmental sounds, and the emotional tone of voice.

She may experience visual or auditory hallucinations even though she is unaware of her surroundings.

She may sleep 20 hours or more per day. She may have seizures, experience difficulty with swallowing and she is at a greater risk for skin infections.

Chapter 7 – The Global Deterioration Scale Characteristics

The last ability she will lose before death will be the ability to smile. This can occur a few months or a few weeks before the process of actively dying begins.

At this final stage, her brain can weigh approximately one pound.

8

Grief

The grieving process is seemingly unending for the families of a person with dementia. Dr. Elisabeth Kubler-Ross is considered the pioneer of grief research. In her work, she divided grief and the processing of grief into five distinct stages. Kubler-Ross described these five stages as denial and isolation, anger, bargaining, depression and acceptance.

The stages of grief can apply to a variety of situations revolving around some type of loss, but Kubler-Ross' research specifically involved the grief process associated with death.

Not everyone will experience all the phases of grief, nor will the stages necessarily follow in the order given by Kubler-Ross. But most people will. The challenge for families of persons with dementia is "The Long Goodbye." The person you love dies a little bit at a time and just

Chapter 8 - Grief

when you think you can grieve no more, Mom enters another stage or declines a bit more.

This is one of the areas about dementia that is hardest for the families. The person is stolen bit by bit and with the physiological changes, the "Four A's," the loss of physical presence, the loss of personality, the excruciatingly slow loss of the person you love, family members tend to revolve through the stages of grief over and over again.

Families go through these stages so often; they sometimes delude themselves into thinking they are ready for the end. But the reality for them is this: even with your grief, even with all the pain and hurt, until death occurs, you can still walk back into that room and see your mother. Death is a final act which will not allow you to do that part again.

When we are told of a loved one's imminent death, we also go into a state of shock or denial. The feelings are related more to sadness and disbelief, without the finality of death.

But when we learn of a loved one's actual death, we go into a deeper type of shock and disbelief. The brain has only present term memories of the deceased person, so it temporarily shuts down and begins to move memories and information to past tense status. The grieving person

Chapter 8 - Grief

may isolate herself during this first stage of grieving. People often report feeling out of touch, they don't necessarily seem aware of their surroundings, they report a feeling of numbness, and some say they don't feel connected to their bodies. They are in shock.

During this initial phase, the person is not really aware of his or her surroundings. The feelings of denial and loss are so severe; he may not be capable of safely driving a car. People often report driving to a place and then not remembering the drive, the red lights, etc. It is safer to let someone else drive you during these first few weeks and months.

Secondly, people tend to experience some type of anger. Anger at the disease, anger that the disease killed their loved one, anger their loved one had the disease. You may be angry at yourself for wishing Mom's death would come and then think somehow you were responsible. (You don't have that kind of power.)

You may be angry that science doesn't know enough about the disease or the doctors were not able to stop the disease process or cure Mom. And honestly, there is anger and fear that with the diseases of dementia, this could happen to you as well.

Chapter 8 - Grief

Currently, there is not enough research to support this fear. Some dementias, like Frontotemporal, do seem to follow a female lineage in the family, but most do not appear to have a traceable hereditary pattern. Studies of identical twins indicate if one twin has Alzheimer's, the other twin has only a 60 per cent chance of also having the disease. And in some families we see one child in ten with the disease and in others we see all ten children getting the disease.

Certainly if your parent has Alzheimer's, your risk goes up 10 – 30 per cent, but to date, that's all we know. One theory at present is Alzheimer's is a virus lying dormant in every human, and for some reason, in some people, it turns on. I talk to a lot of people who insist they know someone whose great-grandmother had Alzheimer's and whose grandmother then had Alzheimer's, etc.

But this would be difficult to prove because when great grandmother and then grandmother "had Alzheimer's" medical science simply didn't have enough knowledge about the disease process of Alzheimer's to be sure. In a normal elderly person, death and aging occur in the home and outside assistance is not needed.

In other words, most people live and die in their own homes. When that happens, when we are faced with the

Chapter 8 - Grief

death of a loved one, Kubler-Ross' stages of grief are encountered again and again.

Thirdly, you are confronted with bargaining. This may involve prayers and offerings to stop this disease or end this disease for the person you love. When interviewed, most people express having these feelings.

Alzheimer's support groups help here because they are for care givers going through the emotional rollercoaster you are riding.

The fourth step we feel is depression. I tell families when I first meet them to be honest with themselves. When they reach a day where they are too exhausted to visit Mom, call instead, or make their visit short. It's important to realize what your limits are and how hard this process is for each family member.

Finally there comes acceptance. Because families cycle through these stages over and over again during the course of the disease process, you may get to acceptance several times and then Mom's condition deteriorates more and you find yourself back at the beginning.

This is why Alzheimer's is referred to as "The Long Goodbye." Families dealing with the disease process may find themselves moving through the stages over and over, going from anger to acceptance and then facing a new

Chapter 8 - Grief

loss of abilities and recognition by their parent, anger and denial, bargaining and depression and finally acceptance again, only to start the process over.

Some spouses and children are unable to deal with the demise and slow loss of their parent or wife. These people arrange for care at a facility and are never seen again. Others face the horror of the disease process daily and continue to stay involved in the life and care of their loved one. Others acknowledge that when they can emotionally and mentally handle the visit, they visit. This may be difficult to understand, but remember what each person is feeling. Some people have unresolved issues and they are trying to find some type of closure. It is no doubt extremely difficult to visit a mother who looks at you with no recognition in her eyes.

I have seen this have a devastating effect on people. Some can't handle it and don't visit. One woman found comfort in her mother only recognizing her as "that nice lady who brings me chocolate." Until you see for yourself the finality of late stage dementia and eminent death, it's tough to judge other family members.

But keep this in mind. Any person, placed at any facility, will automatically get better care the more you

Chapter 8 - Grief

visit. It has nothing to do with the staff; it has to do with human nature.

If you know everyday your boss will check your progress on File A, chances are you will keep File A in tip-top shape. If your boss never checks File B, well you probably keep up with File B, but not as closely.

If the staff knows you visit regularly and observe and watch the interactions of the staff and residents and the care your mom is receiving, then she too will be treated like File A.

And if you are struggling with grief and guilt because you promised Mom you would never place her in a nursing home or an assisted living center then remember this: When you made that promise I'm certain you had no idea your mother would develop this disease.

This is a medical disease, the worst one an aging person and her family can face and it requires 24-hour nursing care. So for medical purposes, she needs placement is a facility that can provide those services.

Questions for you to consider include: Do you continue to visit your mother? Do you continue to honor her place as matriarch of your family? Is she part of your family holidays and celebrations? Do her grandchildren visit and call and send cards? Is her birthday celebrated?

Chapter 8 - Grief

Are you showing your own children that should something happen to you and you should require some type of care like your mother that they are still to honor you?

If you can answer "yes" to these questions, then you have kept your promise to your mother. You have simply had to balance her physical needs with medical care.

Death

I called a woman one time to tell her that if she or her children wanted to say "goodbye" to her husband, their father, they needed to come to the nursing home, because he had only a few days left to live. She thanked me for calling and then said, "No, I don't need to come. My husband died seven years ago and that's just the shell his spirit was in. Our children said their goodbyes several years ago too. Just call me when it's over."

Families react to the pending death of their loved one in a variety of ways. I had a granddaughter come in once when I alerted the family to the fact that the grandmother had begun "actively dying." This granddaughter, who declared she loved her grandmother dearly, had never visited or called her beloved grandmother. She began yelling at the nurse and staff, finally demanding I tell her grandmother to "Stop dying immediately." And she was serious. Unfortunately, I don't have that kind of power.

Chapter 9 - Death

Other families prepare themselves and sit "vigil" with their loved one, day and night. They have made a decision to be there and be a part of this process, to share in the final hours, minutes and breaths. They cry, they laugh, they all say their goodbyes and they are there in the final moments. A difficult time to be certain, but ultimately those days, hours and moments defined them as a family.

Other families only want a call when it's over, so their parent dies with only staff in attendance, or lying in bed all alone as the staff tends to other residents.

Regardless of how the families respond, people die in a somewhat orderly manner. Folks past the age of 70 tend to die within a month of their birthdays, something gerontologists call the "Cycle of Life." The body has used up its resources and it prepares to shut down in a timely fashion, within the season of its birth.

The study of death and dying and its cultural processes is called Thanatology. Cultures and religions view death differently and the United States is no exception. We have a difficult time even saying "dead" in our society. If you read a large city newspaper today, you might be surprised to discover very few people died yesterday. Their obituaries may state the person went "to be a flower" in a

Chapter 9 - Death

garden somewhere far away, or became "an angel" in a choir, or "went home" to see someone, but relatively few people actually died.

We also lack social clues that a person is in mourning. A hundred years ago, a person dressed in black or wearing a certain type of pin would be recognized as a person in mourning or bereavement. Society at large would have given that person deferment for his or her grief time. But even those cultural rules are gone.

We have a fear of aging and death in America and as such we have difficulty mourning our loss or supporting those friends and family members as they mourn. We become frantic when we see people cry and our response it to pat that person on the back and tell him or her "It's okay, it's okay, stop crying."

But the reality is that the grieving person needs to cry. When we mourn or grieve, our brains produce toxins. Grief tears are different than tears formed because I stumped my toe and am in pain.

Grief tears carry the toxins out of the brain produced from grieving. But seeing others cry upsets us, so we want them to stop, but we need to be able to comfort that person and tell them it's okay to cry. Unresolved grief is not healthy, mentally and physically and it will manifest

Chapter 9 - Death

itself in one way or another, either through crying or depression and anger.

You may be afraid to start crying. You may feel if you start you won't be able to stop. Your body needs to cry and when it's finished crying, you will stop. Keep tissue in your car, your purse, at your desk, next to your chair or bed and when you need to cry, do so.

Be prepared that friends and family members may not give you much support. Even good friends or well-meaning church members may give little support. The response may be "You knew your mom was sick," or "You know this is better," or "It's been three months already." The truth is it takes years to mourn the loss of a parent. Ten years is the average mourning time. And it doesn't matter how sick your parent was or how hard it was to be with her near the end of life, she was still your mom, she was still alive. And until her death, you could still walk back into her room and see her, hold her hand, kiss her face.

Family and friends may harbor anger or resentment towards other family members or friends. They may feel one person didn't visit enough or show enough emotion. They may believe a person didn't care. People vary in how they grieve. Someone may be an interactive griever,

Chapter 9 - Death

while another person may be a private griever. A person who can't accept the grieving style of another person may even transfer some anger about the death onto that person.

For the men, they get even less support. After all, they're men, so they don't cry or grieve, right? The truth is men have just as much loss and just as many reasons to cry and they need to cry too. The correct response is to offer a supportive shoulder and hug and simply say, "I'm sorry for your loss."

I know two sisters who sat for seven days with their father as he lay dying. Their husbands had known Dad for 18 years and 25 years respectively. Dad had even lived with one daughter and her husband for several years, until his dementia could no longer be managed at home. His death was mourned by the daughters and the sons-in-law. Their relationships with him had been one of the longest relationships in their lives and he had figured prominently into their lives, as a father figure, grandfather, father-in-law, as another man who enjoyed fishing and hunting. As a father who had no sons, these men filled that void in his life.

Yet when he died, the daughters were viewed differently than their husbands. At the funeral, the

Chapter 9 - Death

daughters were hugged over and over, the sons-in-law were largely overlooked. Yet their grief was just as real.

The Process of Death

The process of death itself is not really a great mystery. If you know the signs to look for, you can see the person preparing to go. And in the final days and hours, the body does very specific things to alert us the end is near. For the most part, the human body ceases function in a way that allows us to track the process and prepare the families.

A few months before death, the person typically becomes more withdrawn. A person with Level Seven dementia will have even greater difficulty swallowing and may begin aspirating on fluids or pureed food. For a while she will be able to tolerate thickened liquids, but eventually the brain damage is so great, she will no longer be able to swallow without the risk of aspirating food or fluid into her lungs. Once a person exhibits great difficulty with chewing, swallowing and eating, that is a signal that the body's gastrointestinal and digestive systems are no longer functioning correctly. Food may be taken in, but the body cannot utilize it. Food is no longer wanted or needed.

Chapter 9 - Death

As the disease advances during this time, your loved one will be even less and less involved or interested in her surroundings. She will continue to have little or no interest in food or hydration and may even fight to avoid being fed, clamping her mouth shut or trying to move her head away from the spoon of food. She appears to go inside herself even more; some see this as the start of a spiritual journey. She will have lost the ability to smile a few weeks or months before her eating stops.

If she is in Level Five or Level Six, several weeks before death, she will become even more withdrawn and start this process. Families often report their mother is no longer looking at them when they visit. Instead she seems to be looking beyond them, to something else. Often they see her reach out, stretch an arm and they watch as her fingers try to grab or touch something in the air they can't see.

Families report hearing their mom or dad talk to people they can't see. One son said he heard his father clearly say in a somewhat agitated voice, "No, not yet, now go away." When the son asked who his dad was talking to, the father pointed to the wall above the son's head and replied, "That woman there. She wants me to go with her

Chapter 9 - Death

and I don't want to go yet." Frank died three days later, after his last child arrived to say goodbye.

The looking past others and reaching out is something people who work with death see frequently. It is a sign that the person is entering into the last week of life. Many people believe it is the person reaching out for the other side, and the talking is to spirits or loved ones already gone, now waiting for her.

This is considered to be the first step of actively dying. Actively dying means a person has reached the point where her body is starting to shut down. The body does this in a very organized manner, starting with reaching out with the hands and looking beyond those present in the room.

The body shuts itself down over a number of days, unless there is a sudden event, such as a heart attack or a stroke. Her body will begin to pull blood back from the extremities – the arms and legs. Families will notice the hands and feet getting cold and then warm, cold and them warm.

After a few days or even hours, the feet and hands will stay cool to the touch and mottling in the hands and feet will begin. Mottling occurs when blood is no longer circulating at a high rate and is now pooling in the

Chapter 9 - Death

extremities. Her skin will have purple or bluish coloring in the feet and hands. The fingernails will become blue. As this progresses, mottling will be seen in the knees and buttocks, as well as the elbows.

The person may begin to have moments of twitching or jerking, known as Pre-Termination Agitation. As the muscles receive less and less oxygen, the cells respond and cause the jerking movement.

Medications can be used at this time to alleviate this spasmodic behavior.

The body is now supplying blood only to the trunk area and the vital organs. Breathing has changed from lung breathing, where the rib cage rises and falls to mouth and abdominal breathing.

The person will be semi-comatose, non-responsive, and she will be breathing through her mouth. Her stomach or abdomen will rise with each breath.

Aspiration risks began about the time breathing changed, so hydration and nutrition are withheld to avoid causing the person to choke to death. This is not the same as if you or I didn't get food or water. The dying person's body can no longer utilize food or water. At this point you will use a dental sponge to keep the mouth and tongue moist.

Chapter 9 - Death

Breathing will be shallow and heavy, and there will probably be a gurgling sound as saliva has pooled in the back of the throat. The person cannot swallow the saliva, and the sound can be upsetting to hear. However, it is not necessarily causing distress to the dying person. There are medications, including a patch, which can be used to help dry up the saliva.

The sound of the gurgling breathing can be very upsetting, so some families want oxygen used. The oxygen will not help the dying person, as she is now breathing through her mouth and her body is no longer utilizing oxygen anyway. The machine is primarily used to make families feel better. The noise helps cover the gurgling sound.

As the person nears death, apnea begins. Apnea is where the person will stop breathing for several seconds at a time and then begin to breathe again. This can be very frightening if you are not ready. Apnea can start and stop for several days, but in the final hours it is constant. In the final minutes, there is more apnea than breathing and finally, one last long breath.

As the person is dying, she will be less and less responsive; finally there will be no response for the last few days or hours. Her eyes may be half open and her

Chapter 9 - Death

mouth will be wide open as she breathes. You may notice the tongue changes color or the back of the mouth changes color, these are normal.

She may or may not respond to your voice or your touch. People who work in the field of death believe persons need to be told they have permission to go on, that is, you actually tell your mom or dad or husband or wife that it's okay to go, even if there doesn't seem to be a response.

By this time the facial features will have relaxed and skin coloring will have changed. She will look very peaceful. The breathing will continue, but respirations will have slowed to between four to10 per minute. The pulse will be thready and the heart beat will be more erratic. Kidney function will have ceased, as the body continues to shut down.

As the person draws a last breath, the body may have a shudder. The bowels and bladder may evacuate. At the end, unlike what we see on television, the mouth and probably the eyes will stay open. This is because the brain no longer functions to send a message to the muscles to shut the eyes or the mouth. And unlike those shows, passing your hand over the eyes will not shut them.

Chapter 9 - Death

If you are not prepared for this, the person can appear to be grimacing or be giving some sign of pain. This is simply not true. With not muscle contracture, the mouth opens and stays open. This is simply what death looks like in reality. It is the normal course of events.

If you are in a facility, the staff will come in to clean the body. If you are using hospice care, then a hospice nurse will arrive to declare death. If not, the nurse in the building will do so. The staff will contact the funeral home and they will send someone to retrieve the body.

And the grief process will begin again, almost as if you had never worked through any of the grief stages. That's because until this moment, you could still be with the person you loved, you could still hold her hand. You could still smell her skin, touch her, and brush her hair, or rub lotion on her hands.

Even with the comfort of spiritual or religious beliefs, this is the most difficult part, because now the person we loved is physically removed from us. We ache in a new way; we feel a void that wasn't there before.

The Brain

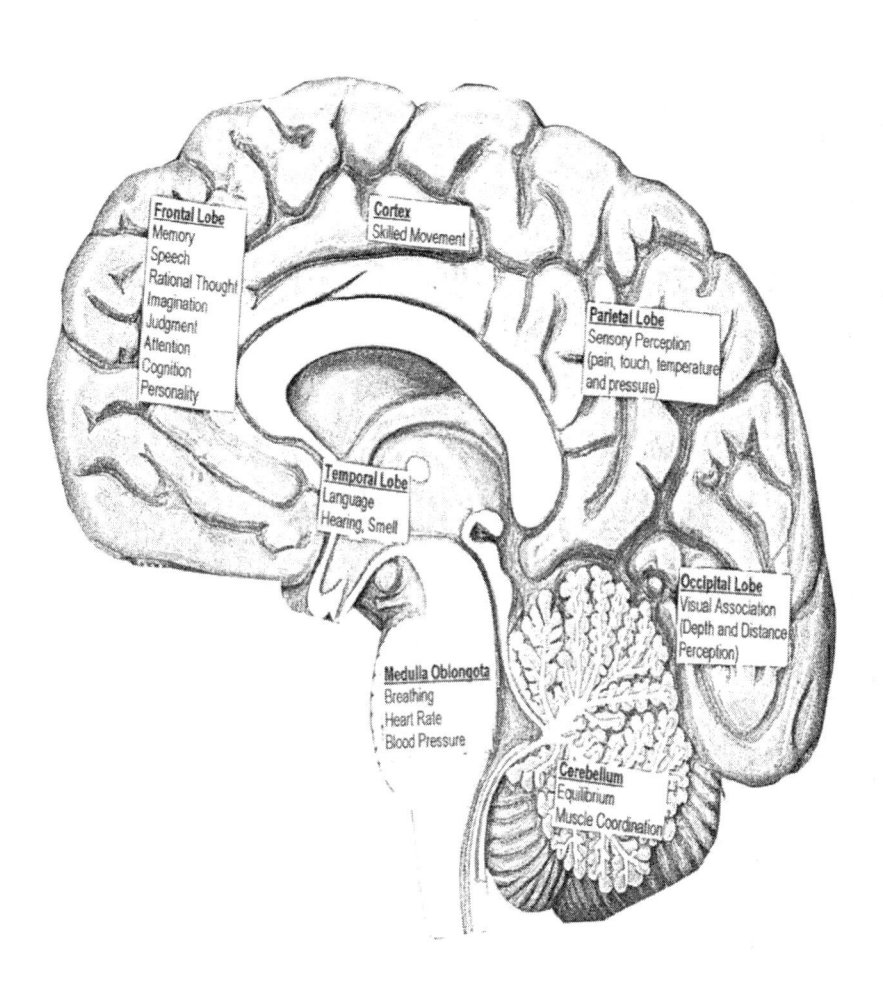

Frontal Lobe
Memory
Speech
Rational Thought
Imagination
Judgment
Attention
Cognition
Personality

Cortex
Skilled Movement

Parietal Lobe
Sensory Perception
(pain, touch, temperature
and pressure)

Temporal Lobe
Language
Hearing, Smell

Occipital Lobe
Visual Association
(Depth and Distance
Perception)

Medulla Oblongota
Breathing
Heart Rate
Blood Pressure

Cerebellum
Equilibrium
Muscle Coordination

Made in the USA
Charleston, SC
25 April 2011